Communication skills for doctors

Best practice guide

∞∞∞∞∞∞∞∞∞∞∞∞∞∞∞

Dr Rajeev Gupta

Consultant Paediatrician

Barnsley Foundation Hospital

Hon Professor, Sir John Hicks College of Economics and management, Leeds, UK

"EVERYTHING THAT IRRITATES US ABOUT OTHERS CAN LEAD US TO AN UNDERSTANDING OF OURSELVES." —CARL JUNG

Contents

Introduction

Effective communication skills are the foundation of success not only socially and personally, but also in business and profession. Communication is essential to the success of a medical consultation and highest patient satisfaction. Doctors or physicians communicate on various fronts all the time and an intuitive awareness of the various components and underpinning principles of communication will give a better control, and perhaps increase efficiency.

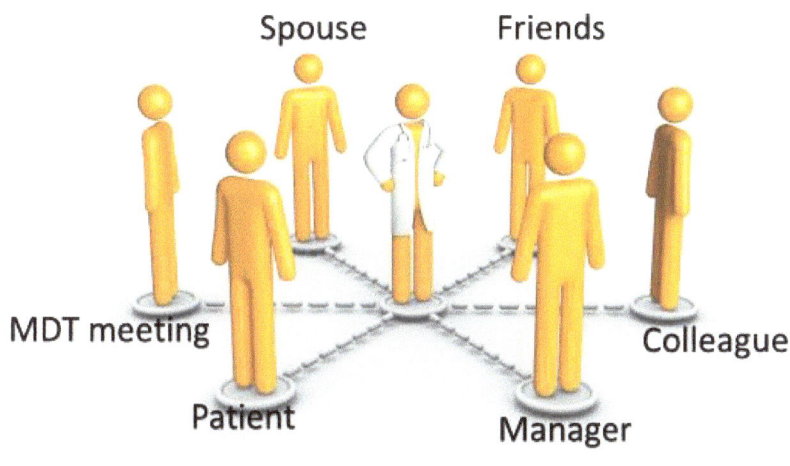

Spouse   Friends

MDT meeting   Colleague

Patient   Manager

Doctor's communication

A good communication results in a better patient satisfaction, positive effect on the overall outcome of patient care; increased compliance and adherence to proposed plans of therapy and a decreased probability of complaints or litigation. Poor communication skills have a negative effect on the overall outcome of patient care.

General medical council mention good communication as essential skill of doctor. Unfortunately, the assumption of good communication skills does not hold true on many occasions and increasing patient expectation risks monitoring of doctor's communication skills. In fact demonstration of good communication skills is a necessary requirement in appraisal and revalidation etc.

Communication is a complex process and the components are not well known to most doctors. A good knowledge of the process and components will give opportunity of a planned and effective communication . What can you recall from your own interaction with your doctor or your dentist? Was it clear? Was it sympathetic? Were your views , concerns and beliefs got explored? Were you left with the impression that you were told as much as you wanted to know? Were you left with the impression that your doctor was a good listener? The answer may possibly be yes and there are good , succinct communicators who effectively convey the message using their verbal and non-verbal skills, you feel comfortable in their company, they listen to you and respect what you say.

Can you think of some one who is not a good communicator? Please jot down why you think he or she is not a good communicator and what could he or she do to get better at it.

…………

……………………

………………………..

………………………………………….

Historically in medicine, there was a paternalistic approach to deciding what should be done for a patient: the physician knew best and the patient accepted the recommendation without question. This era is ending, being replaced with consumerism and the movement toward shared decision-making. Patients are advising each other to "educate yourself and ask questions". Patient satisfaction with their care, rests heavily on how successfully this transition is accomplished. Ready access to quality information and thoughtful patient-doctor discussions is at the fulcrum of this revolution.

We know how often things go wrong in health services. A great majority can be prevented with a good communication. We are living in what has been called the "Communication Age". We are able to communicate information faster, more clearly and more widely than ever before in the history of civilization.

Effective communication is best achieved through simple planning and control; this course will train you at approaches which might help you not only in communication to patients but also day to day conversation to colleagues, family members and friends. It will help you to understand how to communicate your message in the best possible way.

Fundamentals of communication

Making conversation effective

Most conversations sort of drift along and a proportion of it would look wasteful on reflection. To ensure an efficient and effective conversation, there are three considerations:

> ➢ you must make your message understood

> ➢ you must receive/understand the intended message sent to you

> you should exert some control over the flow of the communication

Thus you must learn to listen as well as to speak. If you do not explicitly develop the skill of listening, you may not hear the information / suggestion which may be important.

Many problems that occur in an health care organization are the direct result of people failing to communicate. This may include harm to patient , disputes of colleagues and tension in atmosphere. Faulty communication may lead to confusion and can cause a good plan to fail.

Communication is the exchange and flow of information and ideas from one person to another. It involves a sender transmitting an idea to a receiver. Effective communication occurs only if the receiver understands the exact information or idea that the sender intended to transmit.

Studying the communication process is important because you deal with patients who are inherently vulnerable and depend on you not only to diagnose but also counsel, coordinate, evaluate, and supervise the disease management process.

The Communication Process

Effective communication is all about conveying your messages to other people clearly and unambiguously. It's also about receiving information that others are sending to you, with as little distortion as possible.

Doing this involves effort from both the sender of the message and the receiver. And it's a process that can be fraught with error, with messages muddled by the sender, or misinterpreted by the recipient. When this isn't detected, it can cause tremendous confusion, wasted effort and missed opportunity.

In fact, communication is only successful when both the sender and the receiver understand the same information as a result of the communication.

By successfully getting your message across, you convey your thoughts and ideas effectively. When not successful, the thoughts and ideas that you actually send do not necessarily reflect what you think, causing a communications breakdown and creating roadblocks that stand in the way of your goals – both personally and professionally.

Q. What is your understanding of communication and in your view what are the components of communication?

....

....

....

Components of communication

When we speak face to face , the main components of the process are

> Thought generation: First, information exists in the mind of the sender. This can be a concept, idea, information, or feelings.
> Encoding: Next, a message is sent to a receiver in words, gestures, posture, facial expression, emotions, tone of language or other symbols.
> Decoding: lastly, the receiver translates the words, body language or symbols into a concept or information that he or she can understand.

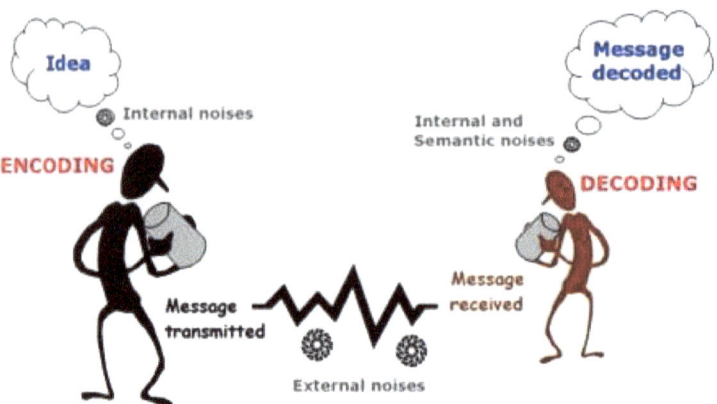

During the transmitting of the message, two elements will be received: content and context.

Content is the actual words or symbols of the message which is known as language - the spoken and written words combined into phrases that make grammatical and semantic sense. We all use and interpret the meanings of words differently, so even simple messages can be misunderstood. And many words have different meanings to confuse the issue even more.

Context is the way the message is delivered and is known as paralanguage - it is the non verbal elements in speech such as the tone of voice, the look in the sender's eyes, body language, hand gestures, and state of emotions (anger, fear, uncertainty, confidence, etc.) that can be detected. Although paralanguage or context often cause messages to be misunderstood as we believe what we see more than what we hear; they are powerful communicators that help us to understand each other. Indeed, we often trust the accuracy of nonverbal behaviours more than verbal behaviours.

The Communications Process

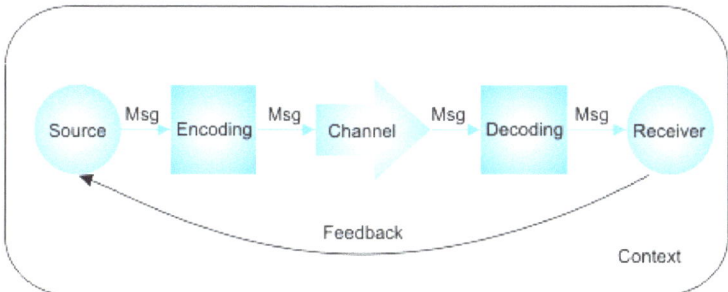

The above flow diagram demonstrates the generation of thought, creation of message, encoding, using a channel like words, body language or e-mail to transmit the message. The right side of the flow diagram corresponds to receiver (listener or reader) who needs to decode the message, interpret it and respond to it based on his or her understanding. This response which can be in form of body posture, muscular tension, facial expression or words becomes a feedback for the sender who may need to modify the further communication based on signals he is getting. This "communication loop" thus continues and paying attention to all components tremendously increases the efficacy of communication. In two way conversation, although the person talking is main sender of message, the person sitting and listening is also emitting body language signals that are being subconsciously received and interpreted by the other person, hence there is constant sending and receiving of message. Increased awareness and sensory acuity will tremendously increase the power of communication.

Some leaders think they have communicated once they told someone to do something, "I don't know why it did not get done. I told Peter to do it." More than likely, peter misunderstood the message. A message has NOT been communicated unless it is understood by the receiver (decoded). How do you know it has been properly received? By two-way communication or feedback as described above. This feedback tells the sender that the receiver understood the message, its level of importance, and what must be done with it. Communication is an exchange, not just a give, as all parties must participate to complete the information exchange.

Handling the components of communication effectively

To be an effective communicator and to get your point across without misunderstanding and confusion, your goal should be to lessen the frequency of problems at each stage of communication process, with clear, concise, accurate, well-planned communications. We follow the process through below:

➤ Source-As the source of the message, *you need to be clear about why you're communicating, and what you want to communicate*. You also need to be confident that the information you're communicating is useful and accurate.

➤ Message-The message is the information that you want to communicate. It is the main element of communication around which the rest of process develops.

9

- Encoding-This is the process of transferring the information you want to communicate into a form that can be sent and correctly decoded at the other end. Your success in encoding depends partly on your ability to convey information clearly and simply, but also on your ability to anticipate and eliminate sources of confusion (for example, cultural issues, mistaken assumptions, and missing information.) A key part of this is knowing your audience i.e. the knowledge and understanding level of the patient, junior doctor or colleague. Failure to understand who you are communicating with will result in delivering messages that are misunderstood.

- Channel-Messages are conveyed through channels, with verbal channels including face-to-face meetings, telephone and videoconferencing; and written channels including letters, emails, memos and reports. Different channels have different strengths and weaknesses. For example, it's not particularly effective to give a long list of instructions for draining a pleural effusion drainage verbally. It needs to be a written procedure to be followed or a demonstration of the procedure.

- Decoding-Just as successful encoding is a skill, so is successful decoding (involving, for example, taking the time to read a message carefully, or listen actively to it.) Just as confusion can arise from errors in encoding, it can also arise from decoding errors. This is particularly the case if the decoder doesn't have enough knowledge to understand the message.

- Receiver-Your message is delivered to individual members of your audience. No doubt, you have in mind the actions or reactions you hope your message will get from this audience. Keep in mind, though, that each of these individuals enters into the communication process with ideas and feelings that will undoubtedly influence their understanding of your message, and their response. To be a successful communicator, you should consider these before delivering your message, and act appropriately.

- Feedback- Your audience will provide you with feedback, as verbal and nonverbal reactions to your communicated message. Pay close attention to these signals, this can give you confidence that your audience (receiver) has understood your message. If you find that there has been a misunderstanding, at least you have the opportunity to send the message a second time.

- Context- The situation in which your message is delivered is the context. This may include the surrounding environment or broader culture (breaking sensitive news, appraisal, research project discussion, presentation to audience etc).

Enhancing Communication effectiveness

Communication is not what is said, but what is received. A poor communication is one of the biggest problems in most organisations and leads to various types of the problems. **People in responsible positions need to constantly improve their communication.** It's not always just what you say. It's also how you "say" it – taking into account your eyes, your posture, your overall body language, even your appearance at the time the communication is exchanged, and the voice in which you offer the exchange make an impact on the person you are talking to.

In verbal communication, an active dialogue is engaged with the use of words. At the same time, however, non-verbal communication takes place, relying on nonverbal cues, such as gestures, eye contact, facial expressions, even clothing and personal space.

Nonverbal cues are very powerful, making it crucial that you pay attention to your actions, as well as the nonverbal cues of those around you. If, during your meeting, participants begin to doodle or chat amongst themselves, they are no longer paying attention to you: Your message has become boring or your delivery is no longer engaging. Patients can grasp when you are thinking something else and not paying attention to what they are saying.

Once again, you need to be mindful of cultural differences when using or interpreting nonverbal cues. For instance, the handshake that is so widely accepted in Western cultures as a greeting or confirmation of a business deal is not accepted in other cultures, and can cause confusion.

While eye contact, facial expressions, posture, gestures, clothing and space are obvious nonverbal communication cues, others strongly influence interpretation of messages, including how the message is delivered. This means paying close attention to your tone of voice, even your voice's overall loudness and its pitch.

Be mindful of your own nonverbal cues, as well as the nonverbal cues of those around you. Keep your messages short and concise. This means preparing in advance whenever possible. And for the impromptu meeting, it means thinking before you speak.

Setting aside and expressing specific time for consultation or meetings increase effectiveness of consultation or meeting.

Enhancing your communications:

- Because gestures can both compliment and contradict your message, be mindful of these.

- Eye contact is an important step in sending and receiving messages. Eye contact can be a signal of interest, a signal of recognition, even a sign of honesty and credibility.

- Closely linked to eye contact are facial expressions, which can reflect attitudes and emotions.

- Posture can also be used to more effectively communicate your message.

- Clothing is important. By dressing for your job, you show respect for the values and conventions of your organization.

- Be mindful of people's personal space when communicating. Do not invade their personal space by getting too close and do not confuse communications by trying to exchange messages from too far away.

Active Listening

Hearing and listening is not the same thing. Hearing is the act of perceiving sound. It is involuntary and simply refers to the reception of aural stimuli. Listening is a selective activity which involves the reception and the interpretation of aural stimuli. It involves decoding the sound into meaning.

Listening is divided into two main categories: passive and active. Passive listening is little more that hearing. It occurs when the receiver of the message has little motivation to listen carefully, such as when listening to music, story telling, television, or when being polite.

People speak at 100 to 175 words per minute (WPM), but they can listen intelligently at 600 to 800 WPM. Since only a part of our mind is paying attention, it is easy to go into mind drift - thinking about other things while listening to someone. The cure for this is active listening - which involves listening with a purpose. It may be to gain information, obtain directions, understand others, solve problems, share interest, see how another person feels, show support, etc. It requires that the listener attends to the words and the feelings of the sender for understanding. It takes the same amount or more energy than speaking. It requires the receiver to hear the various messages, understand the meaning, and then verify the meaning by offering feedback.

Some doctors follow what they saw their consultants doing and seem to believe that the art of medical communication is no different than day to day conversation. While that is a good thinking, it is important to check that their communication is effective, they are giving full benefit to patient or their colleagues including junior doctors and nurses. Miscommunications lead to hazards.

Every patient comes to you with an agenda. Sometimes the agenda is short and simple, sometimes it is lengthy and convoluted. To get to the heart of patient problems and to establish the rapport that is necessary for successful treatment, you may need to artfully explore. Listen to what they are saying and listen to what they are not saying as you take a careful history. **Silence at times tells quite a lot.**

 Remember that you don't really know if the patient is hearing what you have to say, unless you listen to the questions they are asking and the comments they are making. Patients seldom return to doctors who don't take the time to listen to what they have to say.

Videotaped interviews show that doctors interrupt their patients and redirect the communication to areas that they want to learn about in an average of 18 seconds of patient dialogue. It can be frustrating and good practice is to allow them to express their entire agenda before you divert the information flow in another direction.

The following are a few traits of active listeners:

- o Spend more time listening than talking.
- o Do not finish the sentences of others.
- o Are aware of biases. We all have them. We need to control them.
- o Never daydreams or become preoccupied with their own thoughts when others talk.
- o Do not dominate the conversations.
- o Plan responses after the others have finished speaking, NOT while they are speaking.
- o Provide feedback, but do not interrupt incessantly.

- Analyze by looking at all the relevant factors and asking open-ended questions. Walk others through by summarizing.
- Keep conversations on what others say, NOT on what interests them.
- Take brief notes but keep eye contact as much as possible.
- Use paraphrasing to check you have understood the other person correctly.

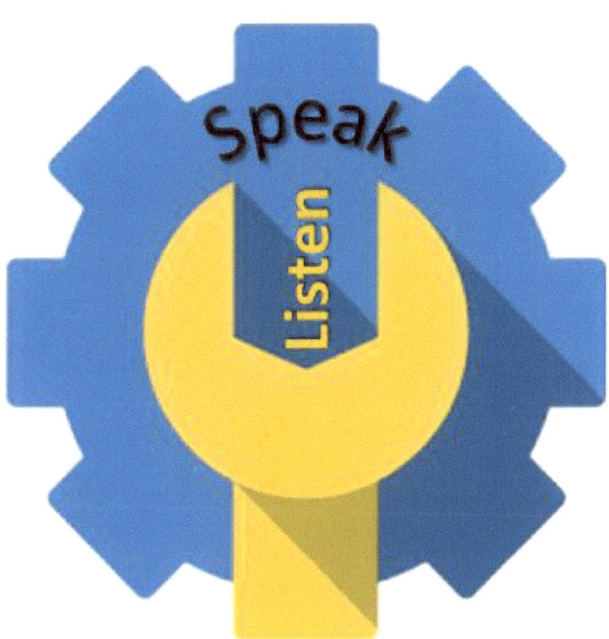

Improving Nonverbal Behaviours

To deliver the full impact of a message, use nonverbal behaviours to raise the channel of interpersonal communication:

- ➤ Eye contact: This helps to regulate the flow of communication. It signals interest in others and increases the speaker's credibility. People who make eye contact open the flow of communication and convey interest, concern, warmth, and credibility.
- ➤ Facial Expressions: Smiling is a powerful cue that transmits happiness, friendliness, warmth, and liking. So, if you smile frequently you will be perceived as more likable, friendly, warm and approachable. Smiling is often contagious and people will react favourably. They will be more comfortable around you and will want to listen more.
- ➤ Gestures: If you fail to gesture while speaking you may be perceived as boring and stiff. A lively speaking style captures the listener's attention, makes the conversation more interesting, and facilitates understanding.

➤ Posture and body orientation: You communicate numerous messages by the way you talk and move. Standing erect and leaning forward communicates to listeners that you are approachable, receptive and friendly. Interpersonal closeness results when you and the listener face each other. Speaking with your back turned or looking at the floor or ceiling should be avoided as it communicates disinterest.

➤ Proximity: Cultural norms dictate a comfortable distance for interaction with others. You should look for signals of discomfort caused by invading the other person's space. Some of these are: rocking, leg swinging, tapping, and gaze aversion.

➤ Vocal: Speaking can signal nonverbal communication when you include such vocal elements as: tone, pitch, rhythm, timbre, loudness, and inflection. For maximum teaching effectiveness, learn to vary these six elements of your voice. One of the major criticisms of many speakers is that they speak in a monotone voice. Listeners perceive this type of speaker as boring and dull.

Speaking Hints

Speak comfortable words! - William Shakespeare

When speaking or trying to explain something, ask the listeners if they are following you.

- Ensure the receiver has a chance to comment or ask questions.
- Try to put yourself in the other person's shoes - consider the feelings of the receiver.
- Be clear about what you say.
- Look at the receiver.
- Make sure your words match your tone and body language (Nonverbal Behaviours).
- Vary your tone and pace.
- Do not be vague, but on the other hand, do not complicate what you are saying with too much detail.
- Do not ignore signs of confusion.

Evaluating communication and feedback

The purpose of feedback is to alter messages so the intention of the original communicator is understood by the second communicator. It includes verbal and nonverbal responses to another person's message. When we are talking, we are constantly having a feedback from the other person which gives u a clue that the other person is understanding what we are saying and which direction we need to take the conversation to. (feedback during communication is different than feedback for appraisal)

Providing feedback is accomplished by paraphrasing the words of the sender. Restate the sender's feelings or ideas in your own words, rather than repeating their words. Your words should be saying, "This is what I understand your feelings to be, am I correct?" It not only includes verbal responses, but also nonverbal ones. Nodding your head or squeezing their hand to show agreement, dipping your eyebrows shows you don't quite understand the meaning of their last phrase, or sucking air in deeply and blowing it hard shows that you are also exasperated with the situation.

Imagine how much better daily communications would be if listeners tried to understand first, before they tried to evaluate what someone is saying.

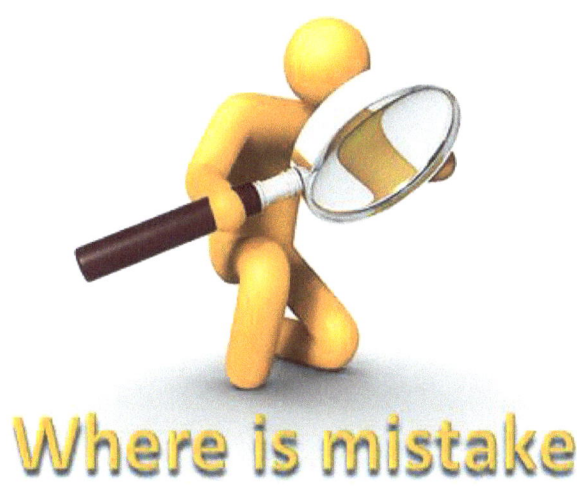

DOCTOR PATIENT CONSULTATION

Communication can be seen as the main ingredient in medical care.

Three different purposes of communication are identified, namely: (a) creating a good inter-personal relationship; (b) exchanging information; and (c) making treatment-related decisions.(Ong LM, de Haes JC, Hoos AM, Lammes FB., Doctor-patient communication: a review of the literature. Soc Sci Med. 1995 Apr;40(7):903-18.)

To be effective, the clinician must gain an understanding of the patient's perspective on his or her illness. Patient concerns can be wide ranging, including fear of death, mutilation, disability; ominous attribution to pain symptoms; distrust of the medical profession; concern about loss of wholeness, role, status, or independence; denial of reality of medical problems; grief; fear of leaving home; and other uniquely personal issues. Patient values, cultures, and preferences need to be explored. Gender is another element that needs to be taken into consideration. Ensuring key issues are verbalized openly is fundamental to effective patient-doctor communication. The clinician should be careful not to be judgmental or scolding because this may rapidly close down communication. Sometimes the patient gains therapeutic benefit just from venting concerns in a safe environment with a caring clinician. Appropriate reassurance or pragmatic suggestions to help with problem solving and setting up a structured plan of action may be an important part of the patient care that is required. Counselling around unhealthy or risky behaviours is an important communication skill that should be part of health care visits. Understanding the psychology of behavioural change and establishing a systematic framework for such interventions, which includes the five As of patient counselling (assess, advise, agree, assist, and arrange) are steps toward ensuring effective patient-doctor communication. (Teutsch C., Patient-doctor communication. Med Clin North Am. 2003 Sep;87(5):1115-45.)

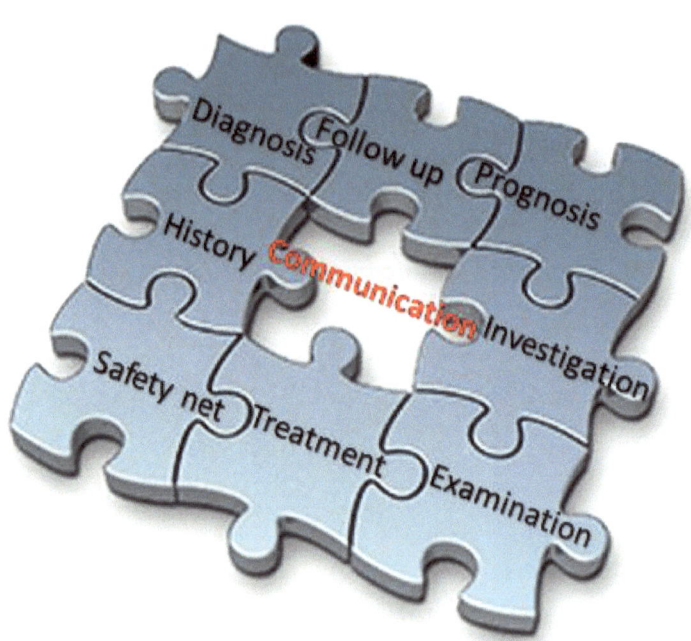

BEST Model of Communication

Consequences of specific physician behaviours are apparent on certain patient outcomes, namely: satisfaction, compliance/adherence to treatment, recall and understanding of information, and health status/psychiatric morbidity.

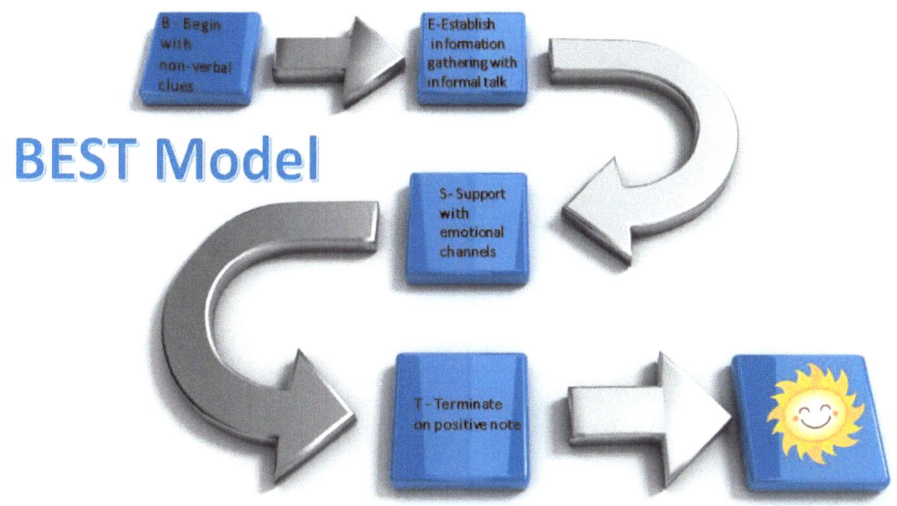

B - Begin with non-verbal clues- First 4 seconds makes most important part of doctor patient consultation, as this is the time to create first impression and sets the direction of thinking. Careful exchange of non-linguistic clues can make the consultation lot more meaningful. Acronym SOFTEN is used to remember sub-components (Smile, Open arm posture, Forward lean, touch with warmth, eye contact, nodding). This acronym is widely used in business world for communication.

In contrast to classical model of doctor –patient communication teaching, BEST model emphasises that the communication does not start with introducing themselves, rather begin lot earlier when doctor first look at the patient in waiting room or at the time of entrance to consultation room. The doctor smiles, and in return the patient smiles. The communication loop is completed. If the patient doesn't smile then it indicates something is going on occupying the mind of the patient and this information is valuable to pitch the consultation. The doctor must try to be neutral to effect of this information, but be mindful of the needs of the patient i.e. this patient may need extra effort to open up or to give emotional support or trust and reassurance.

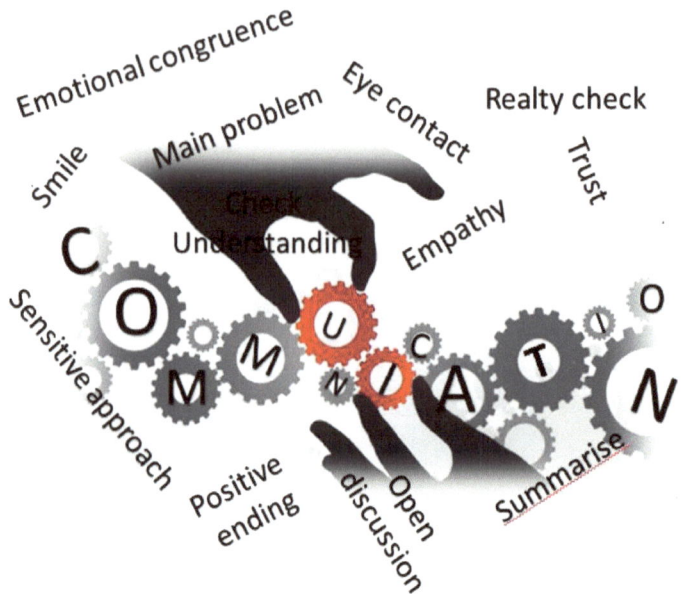

Smile- There is a saying- "Smile is the shortest distance between two people". A rapport can be generated and patient anxiety can be relieved instantly through a smile, hence the doctor should smile at least at the beginning of the consultation unless he/she is breaking bad news. Lot of patients have apprehension when they come for consultation , a gentle smile ease that apprehension, bridge the initial gap and strengthen the relationship between doctor and patient. . Even to unhappy patient, smile gives opportunity for building rapport. "Smile is a curve that sets many things straight" and is said to generate happy hormones and endorphins. We need to try consciously initially and later it will become a natural part of the consultation practice.

Open arm posture helps to show your openness in discussion and encourage patient to tell you more. Clenched fist gives a meaning of frustration and strong aversion. Free hand movements of a doctor in conversation give more confidence to a patient and most patients feel comfortable. Rigid or limited arm posture gives a suspicion that doctor may not be telling the entire story to patient.

Forward lean is a gesture for warmth signifying that you are paying attention. Leaning slightly forward communicates to patient that you are approachable, receptive and friendly.

Touch in form of hand shake is traditional and helps to strengthen a relationship. Hand shake traditionally says a lot about your sincerity and openness to patient and also grasp information about how patient is feeling (skin to skin contact). It is however not necessary to touch physically, doctor need to have ability to greet and engage the patient instantly building the bridge of relationship which is equivalent to touching. Further, it needs to be understood that in certain cultures (i.e. Muslims) physical touch , particularly to ladies may not be appropriate. Touch not only facilitates the sending of the message, but the emotional impact of the message as well. In breaking bad news a tap on shoulder or back of hand helps to strengthen patient's emotions.

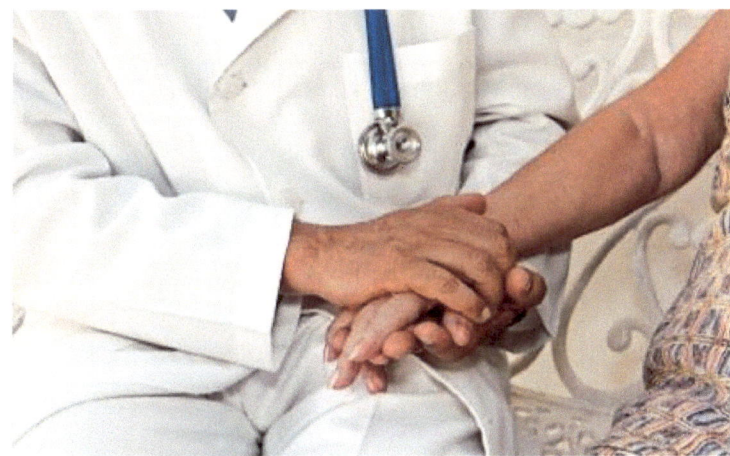

Eye contact is the strongest non-verbal way of communication and allows you to gauge the understanding of patient (if practised correctly). Good eye contact 60-80% of time with in 2 cm of orbital area is considered good and facilitates a good communication. This is specifically important when you are talking as you can listen through eyes (any sign of discomfort or query can be read on patient's face and you can pause to explain it). People rely on visual clues to help them decide on whether to attend to a message or not. If they find that someone isn't 'looking' at them when they are being spoken to, they feel uneasy. Good eye contact make them feel at home and equal. Good eye contact also helps your patient to develop trust in you, thereby helping you and your message appear credible. It can convey emotion, signal when to talk or finish, or hint an aversion. The eye contact has become restricted in recent times due to working on computer in GP consultation and does have an adverse effect. It is however worth remembering that staring can probably be as bad as having no eye contact.

Nodding is encouragement and some patients need it more than others. Nodding is taken as important encouraging clue in body language analysis and understanding of human interaction and communication. It has been found interestingly important on robotic models of human communication.

For both doctor and the patient, images of body language and facial expressions will likely be remembered longer after the consultation than any memory of spoken words.

Doctor must observe patient's non verbal clues, and possibly match or mirror some of these to allow a deeper rapport. Understanding the communication style of patient i.e. visual, auditory or kinaesthetic and acting accordingly will improve the communication greatly (it is used in business world by the business executives and sales persons all the time and does make a difference).

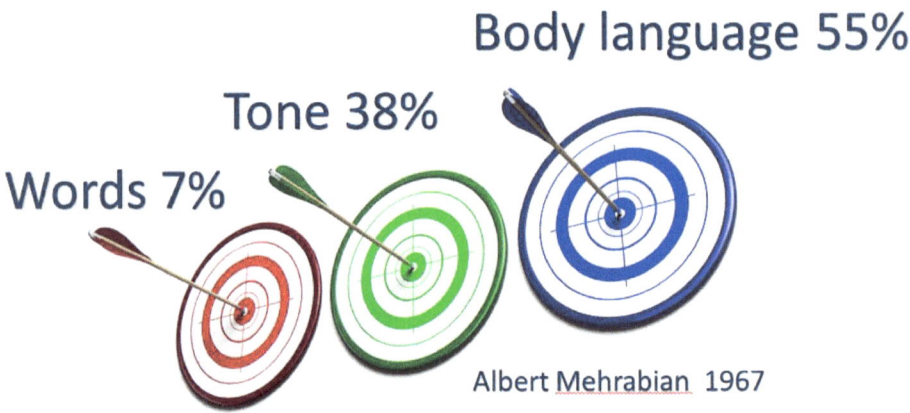

Words 7%   Tone 38%   Body language 55%

Albert Mehrabian 1967

Nonverbal communication is most important because in a study by Albert Mehrabian which is frequently quoted world wide – words convey only 7%, tone 38% and body language 55% of the human communication. In our context, there is evidence that doctors' nonverbal communication abilities are associated with outcomes of medical care such as satisfaction and compliance (*Waitzkin , 1984*) . Doctor's non-verbal communication *(eye-contact, posture, nods, distance, communication of emotion though face and voice)* is positively related to patient satisfaction *(DiMatteo et al 1986, Weinberger et al 1981, Larsen and Smith 1981).*

Tonality of voice constitutes 38% communication and is made up of different elements i.e. pitch, inflection, volume, speed, quality and clarity. The tone of voice is extremely important in the telephonic communication as you miss out body language.

Body Language + Tone of Voice + Words = Total Communication

Silence is the other powerful communicator and it is important for doctor to understand the meaning of silence of patient i.e. lack of interest, unhappiness or deep engagement in thinking etc. The doctor should also use it carefully in conversation to emphasise certain messages. Silence can provide a link between messages but if care is not taken, it can create tension and uneasiness, or sever relationship.

The doctor patient communication involves a two-way exchange of nonverbal information. Patients' facial expressions are often good indicators of what's going on inside, the doctor's body language and facial expression speak volumes to the patient. The doctor who hurriedly enters the examination room several minutes late, takes furious notes, and turns away while the patient is talking, almost certainly conveys impatience and minimal interest in the patient. The patient may interpret such nonverbal behaviour as a message that his or her visit is unimportant, despite any spoken assurances to the contrary (Travaline and Ruchinskas 2005).

E_-Establish information gathering with informal talk- acronym MOGIS (Main problem, Open discussion, Gather other relevant information, Interpretation and provisional diagnosis, Sharing information)

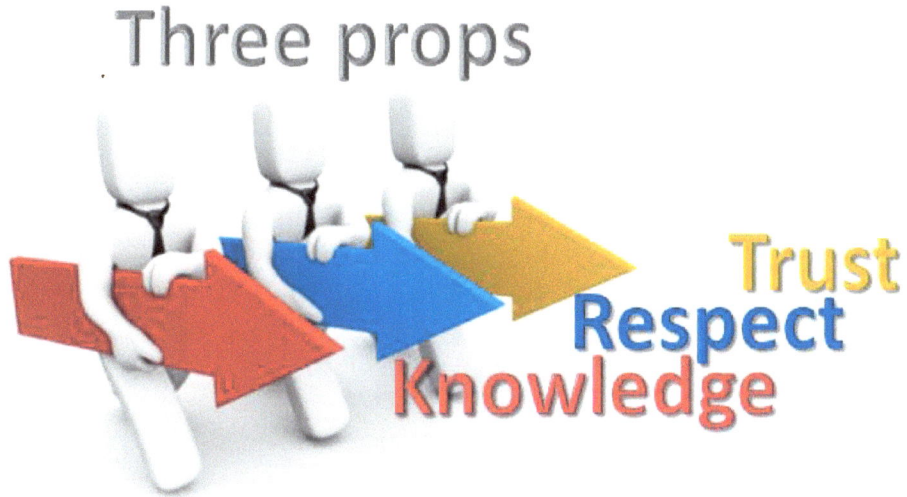

This is main body of consultation and mainly stalks methodology for exchanging information relating to diagnosis. The idea is to gather information from patient to reach a diagnosis and discussing it in a manner desired by the patient. Communication between doctors and patients fails not because patients don't understand what they have been told but because doctors fit what patients say to them into an inappropriately exact medical framework.

Main problem- Asking about main problem in a succinct way is a skill. It has been estimated that doctors interrupt patients within 23 seconds as they try to explain their problems - (Marvel MK et al 1999). In 34 out of 51 visits, the doctor interrupted the patient after the initial concern, apparently assuming that the first complaint was the chief one, 94% of all interruptions concluded with the doctor obtaining the floor.

A study of outpatient visits found that when given the chance to speak uninterrupted at the beginning of the visit, patients required only 93 seconds on average. Eighty percent of all patients stopped talking after two minutes (Langwitz 2002). Studies suggest that patients who were allowed to complete their opening statement without interruption mostly took less than 60 seconds and none took longer than 150 seconds even when encouraged to continue. The earlier the interruption, the less likely to hear more than one complaint and the more likely to have late arising complaints and to miss important complaints. Only 23% of patients completed their opening statement. Allowing the patient to complete the opening statement led to a significant reduction in late arising problems.

The combination of interruptions and multiple concurrent communication tasks between emergency department staff may be the cause of clinical errors, according to Australian research (anonymous- Australian research 2002).

In a randomized controlled trial of 900 patient encounters found that when patients brought in agenda forms and their physicians were educated about them, the visits were only slightly longer - 1.9 minutes on average, however the number of problems addressed per visit increased by 0.5, and patient satisfaction increased(Middleton 2006).

A good way to start is asking a gentle open question, i.e. "what brings you here" or "what do you think is wrong with yourself" rather than "what's your problem".

Open discussion- This is opportunity to expand on the main problem while the patient is still having plenty of opportunity to express. Some times there may be more than one problem and it gives opportunity to identify what patient wants to discuss in today's consultation. Some times patient use presenting problem as a visiting card, a safe way of establishing contact to find out what sort of person the doctor is – how approachable, how sensitive and understanding is the doctor for revealing the real problem (a teenage girl presenting with mild vaginal discharge may really want to discuss whether she is pregnant, a women presenting with breathlessness may want to discuss lump in her breast or a boy with abdominal pain may want to talk about small size of penis). Open discussion without pre-judgement really encourage articulating the real problem and thus saves time in long run.

It is a well known fact that the focus of light determines the value of person and hence in conversation the person having overt control has more satisfaction. Asking a series of closed questions that medical schools used to teach for history interrogation thus may put the patient off. An easy open question after letting main problem flow is " how has it affected you" and it should give the patient ample opportunity to pour out all concern about his problems. Greater "patient centredness" in the interview leads to greater patient satisfaction (Stewart 1984, Arborelius and Bromberg 1992). There are other studies to support discovering and acknowledging patients' expectations improves patient satisfaction (Korsch et al 1968 - paediatrics, Eisenthal and Lazare 1976, Eisenthal et al 1990 - psychiatry).

Doctor needs to have good listening skills and I can remember Dexter Yager's general statement "A good listener win over a good talker every time" (Yager D 2002). Doctor need to carefully observe the patient during conversation, when the patient "light up" (happy experience and use it as trigger for energy flow) and when the shoulders droop (bad experience, explore the cause of pain).

Gather other relevant information – Doctor's agenda in consultation is to dig the relevant information to make the diagnosis. In addition to open and closed questions, leading questions are asked to reveal the diagnostic clues it may be appropriately termed " Guided history". It is important to remember that just asking closed questions for which patient just have to say yes or no or a short punctuated answer doesn't give full satisfaction to the paitent. The trick of the trade is to gather what is needed for the diagnosis without being drawn too much into peripheral matters, inessentials and irrelevancies. It may mean going out of rapport or giving some other subtle body language hints while talking which the conscious mind doesn't understand (is engaged in talking) but the message is passed on to the sub-conscious mind for cutting the story to the pertinent.

Relevant physical examination should be offered if information can be gained from it for helping diagnosis or in some circumstances for patient satisfaction, alternatively it should be explained to patient that you have enough information to make diagnosis without need for examination (may not need to say in words). Investigation should be offered only if needed to complement history and examination for making diagnosis or to further plan the management. Expected time for getting results and how the doctor will approach the patient on getting results, should be explained.

Interpretation and provisional diagnosis- Although it is important to gather the history or information on paper or in mind, the interpretation of the information given by patient should be simultaneous and contemporary to make a clear way through differential diagnostic tree. It will help in asking the crucial questions which will sway the diagnosis in one or other direction. It is an art to associate the symptoms for formulating a diagnosis or syndrome and good clinicians are good at pattern recognition. They have past experience accumulated in form of mental data bank of impressions, and are able to correlate the story of current patient with past experience for deriving tentative diagnosis. However even the doctors with less experience can also selectively elicit the information about relevant parameters in order to increase the discriminatory power. It is a process of mental rehearsal and a proportion of doctors don't go through the process, thus the diagnostic skills don't mature. This model suggests doctors attempting correlation of symptoms, signs and investigations for unifying diagnosis, and bank the information for future use.

Sharing information- It is appropriate sharing information or your thought process with the patient while you are trolling through hypothesis of the provisional or final diagnosis. There is apprehension in mind of a good proportion of doctors that they should hold the information and speak to patient about it only after their mind has digested information to bring up a provisional diagnosis. There is fear in mind of some doctors that the patient will not respect if they don't do so; however it is not true and in our consultation with patients, most patients preferred doctors talking about their interpretation all the way through. The sharing however needs t be tailored to understanding level of patient and in simple lay language. Plain English campaign is good to teach that. Obviously the medical jargon or frightening disease names need to be simplified to help patient understanding. A two way sharing process provides more sense of involvement to patient and is helpful in deciding direction for future management plan.

Doctors have been blamed for being autocratic and self centred rather than patient centred. Regarding the sociolinguistic structure of communication, doctors often maintain a style of high control, which involves many doctor-initiated questions, interruptions, and neglect of patients' "life world." (*Waitzkin , JAMA, 1984)*. Giving the patient the opportunity to discuss their health concerns rather than simply answer closed questions leads to better control of hypertension (Orth et al 1987).

Some times patients have fear of disease and have looked on internet. They watch everything during consultation and allaying their anxiety by talking to them is helpful. Sometimes they bring a list of questions and it's good to acknowledge the importance of list rather than being scared of time consumption in explaining. Scrager and Guard 2009 describe a good 5 step method of dealing with patients who have a list.

Using patient-centred communication to set the agenda for the visit and address the entirety of patients' concerns has been shown to improve not only patient satisfaction but also adherence to treatment recommendations.(Bergeson...and dean 2006, Epstein 2008).

S- Support with emotional channels – This is apparently a part of doctor-patient communication most desired by patients and unfortunately not done well by many doctors. Acronym EERAST is a useful reminder (Empathy, Emotional congruence, Realty check, Attitude of exploration of concerns, Sensitive, caring approach, Trusting attitude).

All human beings are emotionally labile individuals, especially when they are in pain, are ill or are at risk of illness. Uncertainty and fear comes with expectation of illness and almost all patients experience it at some stage.

Empathy- Understanding the patient's feelings and emotions is an art and is a basic skill most doctors develop to some extent. Doctor should recognise emotions in the patients, these emotions need to be acknowledged and further explored during the consultation. Doctors should not ignore or minimize patient feelings with a redirected line of inquiry relentlessly focused on "real" symptoms. Patient satisfaction is likely to be enhanced by doctors who acknowledge patients' expressed emotions (Travaline and Ruchinskas 2005). Doctors who do this are less likely to be viewed as uncaring by their patients (Suchman 1997).

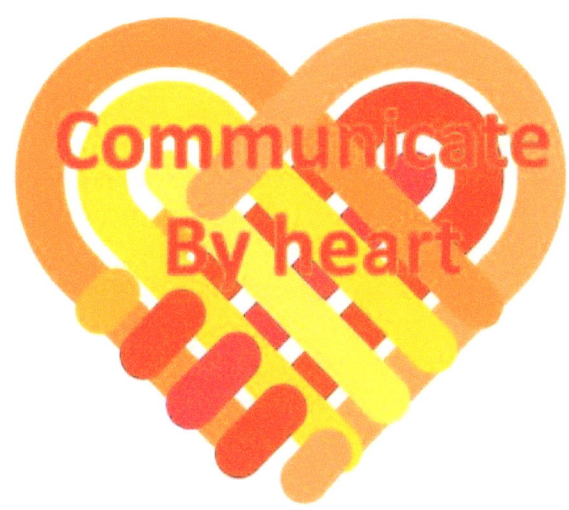

Caring doctors support the patient in expression of feelings, perceptions and beliefs. Doctor's consultation should not be stereotyped, but based on emotional understanding of the patient. Discovering patients' expectations leads to greater patient adherence to plans made whether or not those expectations are met by the doctor (Eisenthal and Lazare 1976, Eisenthal et al 1990). Korsch et al's seminal study in 1968 of 800 visits to paediatric walk-in outpatients in Los Angeles was the first research to tackle the doctor-patient interaction using rigorous methods and doctor's lack of warmth and friendliness was one of the most important variables related to poor levels of patient satisfaction and compliance.

Emotional congruence- Doctor should not only be able to understand patient's perspective but should also be able to give support with his/her emotions. Most people who are unwell, look to the doctor for emotional reassurance in addition to advice and treatment. There is a Chinese proverb - "Words are just words and without heart they have no meaning". Support the conversation with emotional channels, listen the unsaid, feel the feelings of patient and transmit the message from heart to heart, allowing non-verbal two way communication. "People like people like themselves" meaning thereby that if you are on the same planet of thinking and understanding as they are, patient will understand and follow your instructions more vigorously. It is an art and will develop if you are keen and sincere for welfare of the patient. Value of empathy and emotional congruence in breaking bad news is immense.

It is important to recognize that the doctor-patient encounter involves a two-way exchange of nonverbal information. Patients' facial expressions are often good indicators of sadness, worry, or anxiety. The doctor who responds with appropriate concern to these nonverbal cues will likely impact the patient's illness to a greater degree than the doctor wanting to strictly convey factual information (Travaline and Ruchinskas 2005).

Although we knew physicians' communication style and perceptions affect outcomes, few studies have examined how these perceptions relate to the way physicians communicate with patients. Richard et al 2007 have reported that physicians displayed more patient-centred communication and more favourably perceived patients who expressed positive affect, were more involved, and who were less contentious.

Realty check – While it is vital to pay attention to patient's emotions, it is unwise to lose the touch with the facts. Doctor shouldn't fly in emotions although he/she should respect and respond to the emotions of the patient or the relative. Assertion for the contrary with evidence is quite useful if the doctor think there are unfounded fears in the patient or relative's mind. The key is "Question skilfully and listen carefully". An example is "Although you think your child is not eating for past 3 months, his weight is appropriate for age and according to growth chart it has stayed appropriate for past 3 months which indicates that he is getting what he needs; what's your view".

Showing parents that growth chart will probably be the biggest reassurance to them, even in anxious state and most useful part of consultation from their point of view, as said to me by a parent in personal experience. It helps clarifying the perception of the patients if they are overplaying or underplaying the illness, through objective questions and findings of examination or investigations.

It is also important that the doctor is not judgemental. In a qualitative research on osteoporosis, it was revealed that doctors were visually profiling women who they thought would not accept a self-injected treatment based on how fragile the woman looked (Nelson 2009)

Attitude of exploration of concerns – Patients come to doctors with different reasons and different expectations. Some expect the doctor to quickly examine and reassure there is nothing wrong, others want him to write a prescription. There are some others who want specific issue to be addressed and have a reassurance i.e. they don't have a cancer or they don't need operation etc. There is another group which expect doctor to say that the symptoms they are experiencing are real although it may be a psychosomatic illness. Yet another group might like a reassurance that "it is not going to become worse according to my experience" or "we need to operate now else it may become worse". There are others who want to discuss all diagnostic possibilities as they researched on internet. In general practice an acronym "ICE" is used to remind exploration of *ideas, concerns and expectations*. Doctors can increase adherence to treatment regimens by explicitly asking patients about knowledge, beliefs, concerns and attitudes to their own illness (Inui et al 1976, Maiman et al 1988). Doctor's attitude should be focused on patient's needs and it means digging skilfully the underlying belief and reason for visit/ consultation. Once the discussion on real need is embarked, satisfaction breeds and rest of consultation just glides through. Doctor however needs to be aware of his limitation and should express it clearly, so as to allow meeting the expectation of both the patient and the doctor.

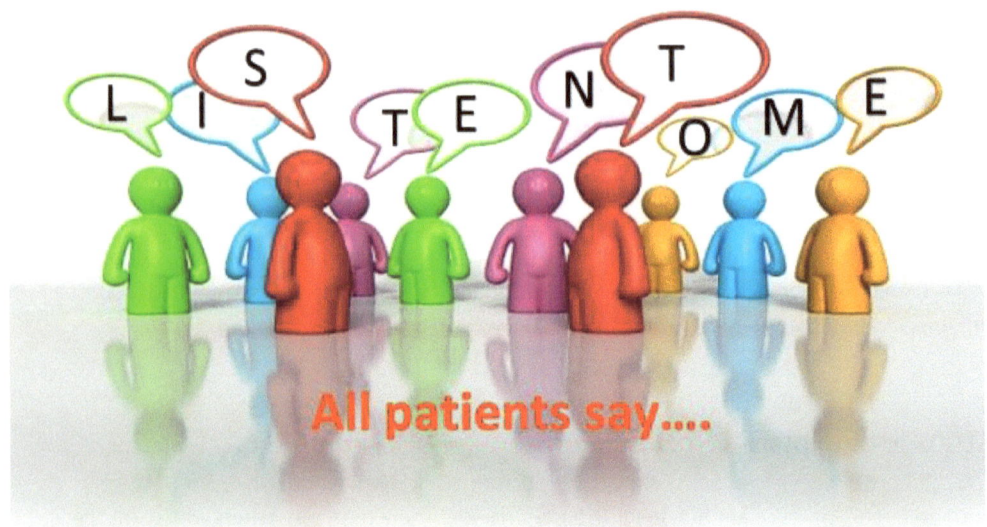

Some questions that can be asked to explore are : What is going on in your life? How do you feel about that? What troubles you about that? How are you handling that? These tend to put patient at ease to express concerns and feel more satisfied with the consultation.

Sensitive, caring approach- Some doctors can give comfort just by talking. They make it easy for patient to talk about uncomfortable topics or situations. There are other doctors who ask questions that may put the patient in discomfort or distress, probably unintentionally. This is either due to a nippy visit from doctor or the doctor in consultation being unable to understand patient's feelings or need. Anecdotally surgeons are blamed for this more often than others. Reading body language and responding to it with your own body language puts the patient's mind at rest without saying words. It is the approach that matters, not the words. You might have heard "I don't care how much the doctor knows until I know how much he cares". The doctor must avoid paternalistic approach at all cost. A careful sensitive listening is all what some patients need and they will thank the doctor for being so helpful.

Breaking bad news is always a very skilled job and needs to be done extremely carefully. Two topics which particularly need tender sensitive approach are death and sexuality. There might be inhibition or reluctance in both doctors and patients to engage in discussion around these areas as there is lack of idea of expectation of the other and a risk of hurting feelings. Carefully designed questions beginning with " Is there any thing you wish to discuss about………" gives an invitation to open discussion in the area and you can carefully deepen the discussion as needed.

Talking to people with a different cultural background or physical , mental or emotional disability etc may need extra care on part of doctor to not make them feel disrespected.

Trust factor – Doctor must have a trusting attitude. A distrust is sensed quickly by the patient and in some way ends the doctor-patient relationship. If you trust patient, through law of reciprocity, the patient trusts you. A doctor who has gone through above phase of empathy, emotional congruence and sensitive caring approach etc develops "unconditional trust factor" (UTF) in the mind of the patient. This means that the patient has enormous trust in what doctor says. This is extremely useful in treatment compliance. Furthermore, this allows human errors of the doctor to be ignored by the patient and we have heard that the patients have chosen not to complain in face of medical errors. Rapport, confidence and trust are necessary in addition to clear grasp of doctor's instructions, for compliance and following specific recommendation (Myerscough 1992). Trust factor also works well when complex situations of ethical dilemma regarding treatment arise. More commonly, trust factor plays extremely important role in consent. It is the job of the doctor to clearly explain risks associated with operation or anaesthesia etc which can be frightening but the confidence and trust in doctor overrides the fear.

You do not want your patients to say: he shows no concern, no warmth, would not answer questions, could not listen The traditional doctor gathers the facts, but the clinician in this age must also discover the patient's own perception regarding their health and lifestyle habits(Steven Eastaw 2004).

EMOTIONAL INTELLIGENCE is overall ability to understand emotions and dynamically react to people and environment, for maximum effectiveness. It extremely important for doctors, however, not much attention is being paid to it at present. It is being recognized as major determinant of success in businesses world due to direct assessment of effect; however, medical field has neglected use of assessment of emotional intelligence for determining the ability of doctor to provide holistic patient care. This is an excellent add-on ability to the technical ability of a doctor and we recommend formal training of all health staff.

T - Terminate on positive note- SECA (Summarise consultation, End with positive comment, Check patient's understanding, Ask if any other issues).

The consultation must end with a sort of conclusion from the doctor whereby the doctor summarise his/her assessment and outlines the proposed treatment . Fletcher called it exposition (Fletcher 1980) and it is fundamental to bring the consultation to a natural end this way, leaving patient with maximum reassurance.

Summarise consultation- It is at times difficult for patients to remember what was being discussed in the flow of conversation and what was the final outcome. Patients may not be bold enough to ask it. Summarising consultation significantly increase retention and compliance. Kupset et al (1975) demonstrated increased in immediate recall of information from 76 to 90% when information was repeated by doctor and the advantage of repetition persisted in postal survey after a month. Ley et al (1973) mentioned clinician to give information category by category i.e. " Now I am going to tell you; what is wrong with you; what tests and investigations will be necessary; what the treatment will be; what you must do to help yourself get better; and what outcome will be." In a study by Ley et al(….) in general practice the recall increased from 50 to 64percent when explicit categorisation was used. Fletcher called it exposition whereby doctor and patient come to end….

End with positive comment as far as possible. If you have carefully listened and thought through out the consultation , you will find few positive points to communicate at the end i.e. "you are so good at understanding all the issues that you will get through it all easy", "you have added advantage of your daughter and other close relatives taking care of you", "the treatment of leukaemia is so much better now that a significant proportion gets disease free life", "your disease is quite complicated but it has been studied quite well- if you had this disease 20 years ago , we will not be able to diagnose it" , "although there is not a lot in terms of treatment, we at least know the diagnosis and that will allow you to know about the usual course of the disease, we know at least it is not cancer which was one of the possibility initially", "although it is a nasty tumour , the good news is that it hasn't had chance to spread yet and chemotherapy will take effect soon", "although your tumour has gone to lungs it is a tiny part affected and chemotherapy is very effective", "you have a prostatic tumour diagnosed on the screening blood test and that is in some way good news as the treatment can control it while if it would have not opted for this test, symptoms would develop much later and treatment is not as effective at that stage", "although your child has Down's syndrome, it is one of the best chromosomal abnormality as many of these children live to happy adult life", "you have a nasty infection however the good news is that it can be cured with antibiotics", . The idea is to change the focus , patient remembers what you told at the end. The patient will remember what you told bad as *we human beings are generally good at noting bad news and not so good at positive news. We don't take much notice of the good news else the television programmes will be full of good news rather than sensational bad news.*

However we need to be realistic to tell the problems rather than ignoring these.

Check patient's understanding- There have been many studies of what patients remember and understand of doctors' explanations. The results, for the most part, are disturbing. Patients' recollections of what was said are hazy, and they don't have much grasp of the risks associated with the treatment offered. (Martyn C 2009 BMJ).

Asking patients to repeat in their own words what they understood of the information they have just been given, increases their retention of that information by nearly 30% (Bertakis 1977). It is clear that patients do not recall all that we impart nor do they make sense of difficult messages. Original studies showed that only 50 to 60% of information given is recalled. Later studies have suggested that in fact much more is remembered and that the real difficulty is that patients do not always understand the meaning of key messages nor are they necessarily committed to the doctor's view. Patient recall is increased by categorisation, signposting, summarising, repetition, clarity and use of diagrams (Ley 1988) . It is at times difficult to ask patient to repeat the information, however a good attention to patient's body language through out consultation and stopping to clarify the point whenever a changed body signal is identified, is a way out for such situation.

One effective way to assess whether the patient is understanding the information is the nature of the questions patients ask; if questions reflect comprehension of the information just presented, a further level of detail may be warranted. If questions reflect confusion, it is advisable that the doctor return to basic information. If the patient has no questions or is obviously uncomfortable, this is a good opportunity for the doctor to stop the discussion, ask explicitly how much information the patient desires, and adjust accordingly (Travaline and Ruchinskas 2005).

Ask if any other issues- Giving other opportunity to bring out any other issues at the end of consultation is extremely important to conclude the consultation to patient's satisfaction, giving all opportunity to say. It may sound bit dodgy as you may open can of worms with this comment, but this may surprisingly bring out the main underlying issue. The patient may not know this as the main problem or knew but wasn't bold enough to express it at the beginning (more effective you are, easier will be for you to bring it out early in consultation). Due to constraint of time you may not be able to address it in this consultation and you may frankly say that you will discuss in next consultation. It is lot better than not addressing it at all and in many occasions the patient understand and address the problem himself/herself once it is spelled out loud. It also gives opportunity to patient for asking what possibly was told by the doctor but was missed or not clearly understood by the patient. It is a good practice any way.

There is decreased understanding of information given if the patient's and doctor's explanatory frameworks are at odds and if this is not discovered and addressed during the interview (Tuckett et al 1985).

In a comparative study of doctors for malpractice claims, several specific behaviours distinguished the no-claims from the claims physicians. No-claims physicians used more statements of orientation (educating a patient about what to expect), laughed and used humour more, and solicited patients' opinions, checked understanding, and encouraged patients to talk more than did claims doctors. No-claims physicians made statements such as "Tell me more about that", or asked patients questions such as "What do you think about taking these pills?". This allowed patients to talk and indicated the physician's interest in their opinions, confirming studies that indicate the importance of allowing patients to talk without interruption (Macready Norra 1997).

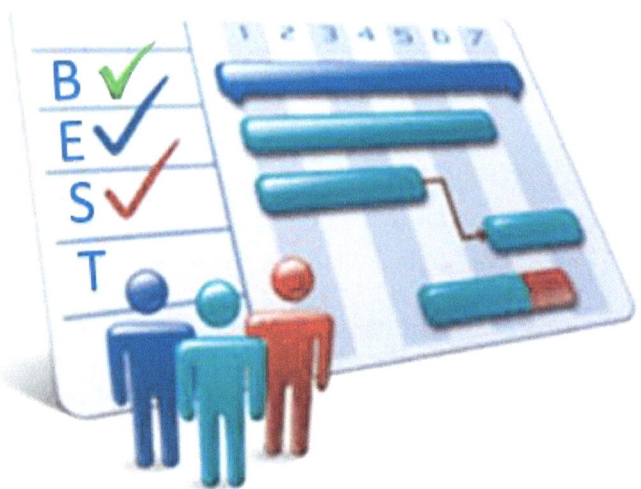

There are some questions the doctor needs to ask himself/herself after each consultation: (RCGP)

Do I know significantly more about this person as a human being than before they came through the door? Was I curious? Did I listen?

Did I explore their beliefs? Did I make an acceptable working diagnosis?

Did I use their beliefs when I started explaining? Did I share options for investigations or treatment? Did I share in decision-making?

Did I make some attempt to see that my patient understood?

Did I develop the relationship (professional, not personal)?

Doctor should attempt to identify personal barriers to communication and learn how can he help patients in narrating story in short succinct way for reaching the appropriate diagnosis and steps of management. Good communication of a doctor will not only benefit patient but also their colleagues in the work environment as well as family and friends. Each person has personal style of communication which is individual, so please keep that style and add whatever you can, to enhance the effect of communication. In a recent article Elizabeth gates mentioned distraction in general practice by physical barriers such as fatigue or stress, or by psychological barriers such as not liking the patient or feeling they have gone over the same ground before.

The most common cause of malpractice suits is failed communication with the patients and their families (Steven eastlaugh 2004). *Body language speaks loudly, more than most doctors realise.* Some non-verbal clues to avoid are- tapping fingers, pens, pencils ; clenching fists ;yawning ; looking out the window ; tapping feet ; crossing arms or legs ; shifting weight from one foot to another etc. These have adverse effect on patient's ability to communicate and can be annoying. Nonverbal communication is to be used to make patient more comfortable.

With pressure from managed care and the resulting demands on medical practices, healthcare professionals are torn between a desire to give the best care possible and their daily race against the clock (Nelson 2009). Even among those who understand the value of communication, a question is often asked – "Does proper communication takes more time"? The answer is, possibly yes initially, but not in long term. John Skelton, professor of communication once said that if you get trained in good communication skills, more effective communication happens and more messages can be passed in shorter time. I would say "Save time by making time to learn the art of communication". In a study in US, Internal medicine residents and doctors taught these skills and those of agenda setting, elicited more of the patients' concerns and allowed more patient talking time without an increase in the length of the visit (Joos et al 1996, Putnam 1988). A busy doctor, a worried patient, and the use of unfamiliar medical terms can lead to confusion and misunderstanding on the patient's part and may sow the seeds for a future malpractice claim. Using a model of communication can help keeping the risk of litigation low even in taxing situations.

There are three outcomes expected from good doctor patient communication – cognitive outcomes i.e. transference of information and knowledge to patient; affective outcome i.e. improved emotional state; behavioural outcome i.e. changed behaviour and habits such as doing exercise, drug compliance etc. The BEST model of communication serves to get the best of all three outcomes in best possible way and yet it is practical and simple to be applied in day to day consultation. It fulfils the medico-social as well as psycho-behavioural aspects of consultation requirements and provides contentment to patients for lasting doctor patient relationship.

Preventing miscommunication

Anything that prevents understanding of the message is a barrier to communication. To deliver your messages effectively, you must commit to breaking down the barriers that exist within each of these stages of the communication process.

Let's begin with the message itself. If your message is too lengthy, disorganized, or contains errors, you can expect the message to be misunderstood and misinterpreted. Use of poor verbal and body language can also confuse the message.

Barriers in context tend to stem from senders offering too much information too fast. When in doubt here, less is oftentimes more. It is best to be mindful of the demands on other people's time, especially in today's ultra-busy society.

Once you understand this, you need to work to understand your audience's culture, making sure you can converse and deliver your message to people of different backgrounds and cultures within your own organization, in your country and even abroad.

Q. What barriers to communication have you come across in your professional or personal life and how did you handle those?

....

....

....

....

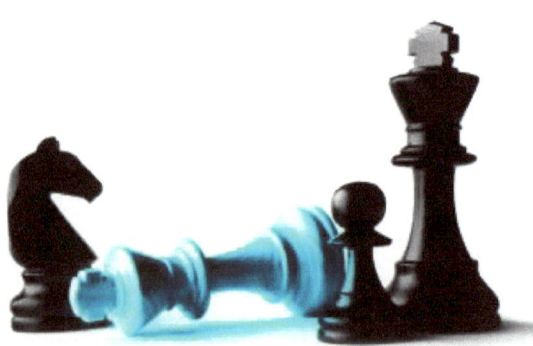

Barriers to communication

There are many subtle physical and psychological barriers to communication that we need to be aware of and need to handle carefully.

- Culture, background, and bias - We allow our past experiences to change the meaning of the message. Our culture, background, and bias can be good as they allow us to use our past experiences to understand something new, it is when they change the meaning of the message that they interfere with the communication process.
- Noise - Equipment or environmental noise impedes clear communication. The sender and the receiver must both be able to concentrate on the messages being sent to each other.
- Ourselves - Focusing on ourselves, rather than the other person can lead to confusion and conflict. The "Me Generation" is out when it comes to effective communication. Some of the factors that cause this are defensiveness (we feel someone is attacking us), superiority (we feel we know more that the other), and ego (we feel we are the centre of the activity).
- Perception - If we feel the person is talking too fast, not fluently, does not articulate clearly, etc., we may dismiss the person. Also our preconceived attitudes affect our ability to listen. We listen uncritically to persons of high status and dismiss those of low status.
- Message - Distractions happen when we focus on the facts rather than the idea. Our educational institutions reinforce this with tests and questions. Semantic distractions occur when a word is used differently than you prefer. For example, the word chairman instead of chairperson, may cause you to focus on the word and not the message.
- Environmental - Bright lights, an attractive person, unusual sights, or any other stimulus provides a potential distraction.
- Smothering - We take it for granted that the impulse to send useful information is automatic. Not true! Too often we believe that certain information has no value to others or they are already aware of the facts.
- Stress - People do not see things the same way when under stress. What we see and believe at a given moment is influenced by our psychological frames of references - our beliefs, values, knowledge, experiences, and goals.

These barriers can be thought of as filters, that is, the message leaves the sender, goes through the above filters, and is then heard by the receiver. These filters muffle the message. And the way to overcome filters is through active listening and feedback.

Barriers of doctor patient communication

Barriers of doctor patient communication may lie in the patients or the doctors (more often than thought generally, becomes quite obvious on reflection of a video recording of the consultation). The other barriers mentioned above still play a role.

A) Barriers within patients and their families:
  a. Lengthy non-directional conversation causing loss of interest of doctor is not unusual (this is how it appears to doctor but it may have a purpose for the patient). Doctor needs to try funnelling the questions to get the useful information.
  b. Shyness, confusion, and fear of death or disability may become a barrier listening to what is said by the doctor. Doctor need to recognise these signals, and allay anxiety honestly explaining the facts.
  c. Information obtained from the Internet and the news media may frequently confuse patients and cause them to have difficulty hearing your message.

    d. Sometimes patients and their families are simply unable to accept bad news. In these cases a second appointment is desirable.

B) Barriers in doctors :

    a. Doctors pursue their agenda i.e. diagnosis and management , not paying attention to patient's concerns

    b. Some doctors try to dominate the conversation and lack good communication skills.

    c. Limitation of consultation time is a barrier in many situations.

    d. Thinking about previous patient which has been puzzling or unusual, may cause lack of concentration of doctor. It is unfair to patient and it is advisable to clear head in such situation with a small break.

    e. Some times a previous experience of a time-waster, anxious or unhappy patient limit the ability of doctor to listen carefully.

    f. Some times doctors tend to anticipate a disagreeable response from patients or their family, and in order to avoid this they present a confusing picture of the patient's condition and prognosis. It is not a good practice and doctor need to be honest and polite.

    g. Some physicians fear the medico-legal consequences to convey the probability of a negative outcome causes them to feel powerless and vulnerable and results in communication that is less than candid.

Keeping the patient focus and patient benefit as prime agenda tend to alleviate many of these barriers.

How to avoid miscommunication

As a doctor (concerned with getting things done) your view of words should be pragmatic rather than philosophical. Thus, words mean not what the dictionary says they do but rather what the speaker intended.

Suppose your manager gives to you an instruction which contains an ambiguity which neither of you notice and which results in you producing entirely the wrong product. Who is at fault? The answer must be: who cares? Your time has been wasted, the needed product is delayed (or dead); attributing blame may be a satisfying (or defensive) exercise but it does not address the problem. In everything you say or hear, you must look out for possible misunderstanding and clarify the ambiguity.

The greatest source of difficulty is that words often have different meanings depending upon context and/or culture. Thus, a "dry" country lacks either water or alcohol; "suspenders" keep up either stockings or trousers (pants); a "funny" meeting is either humorous or disconcerting; a "couple" is either a few or exactly two. If you recognize that there is a potential misunderstanding, you must stop the conversation and ask for the valid interpretation.

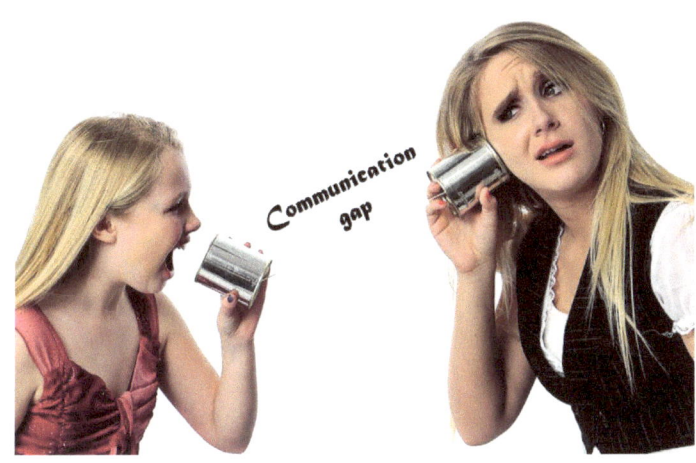

Communication gap

A second problem is that some people simply make mistakes. Your job is not simply to spot ambiguities but also to counter inconsistencies. Thus if I now advocate that the wise manager should seek out (perhaps humorous) books on entomology (creepy crawlies) you would deduce that the word should have been etymology. More usual, however, is that in thinking over several alternatives you may suffer a momentary confusion and say one of them while meaning another. There are good scientific reasons (to do with the associative nature of the brain) why this happens, you have to be aware of the potential problem and counter for it.

Finally, of course, you may simply mishear. The omission of a simple word could be devastating. For instance, how long would you last as an explosives engineer if you failed to hear a simple negative in: "whatever happens next you must [not] cut the blue wi..."?

So, the problem is this: the word has multiple meanings, it might not be the one intended, and you may have misheard it in the first place - how do you know what the speaker meant?

Rule 1: PLAY BACK for confirmation

Simple, you ask for confirmation. You say "let me see if I have understood correctly, you are saying that ..." and you rephrase what the speaker said. If this "play back" version is acknowledged as being correct by the original speaker, then you have a greater degree of confidence in you own understanding. For any viewpoint/message/decision, there should be a clear, concise and verified statement of what was said; without this someone will get it wrong.

Rule 2: WRITE BACK for confidence

But do not stop there. If your time and effort depend upon it, you should write it down and send it to everyone involved as a double check. This has several advantages:

Further clarification - is this what you thought we agreed?

Consistency check - the act of writing may highlight defects/omissions

A formal stage - a statement of the accepted position provides a spring board from which to proceed

Evidence - hindsight often blurs previous ignorance and people often fail to recall their previous errors

<u>Rule 3: GIVE Background for context</u>

When speaking yourself, you can often counter for possible problems by adding information, and so providing a broader context in which your words can be understood. Thus, there is less scope for alternative interpretations since fewer are consistent. When others are speaking, you should deliberately ask questions yourself to establish the context in which they are thinking. When others are speaking, you should deliberately ask questions yourself to establish the context in which they are thinking.

PRACTICAL POINTS

As with all effective communication, you should decide (in advance) on the purpose of the conversation and the plan for achieving it. There is no alternative to this. Some people are proficient at "thinking on their feet" - but this is generally because they already have clear understanding of the context and their own goals. You have to plan; however, the following are a few techniques to help the conversation along.

Assertiveness

Assertiveness is quite important for clarity and effectiveness of communication. The definition of to assert is: "to declare; state clearly". This is your aim. If someone argues against you, even loses their temper, you should be quietly assertive. Much has been written to preach this simple fact and commonly the final message is a three-fold plan of action:

1. acknowledge what is being said by showing an understanding of the position, or by simply replaying it (a polite way of saying "I heard you already")

2. state your own point of view clearly and concisely with perhaps a bit of supporting evidence

3. state what you want to happen next (move it forward)

Thus if you have a time pressure but you are busy you can say "Yes, I see why you need the report by tomorrow; however, I have no time today to prepare the document because I am in a meeting with a customer this afternoon; either I could give you the raw data and you could work on it yourself, or you could make do with the interim report from last week".

You will have to make many personal judgement calls when being assertive. There will certainly be times when a bit of quiet force from you will win the day but there will be times when this will get nowhere, particularly with more senior (and unenlightened) management. In the latter case, you must agree to abide by the decision of the senior manager but you should make your objection (and reasons) clearly known. For yourself, always be aware that your subordinates might be right when they disagree with you and if events prove them so, acknowledge that fact gracefully.

Communicating in complex situations and confrontations

<u>Confrontations</u>

When you have a difficult encounter, be professional, do not lose your self-control because, simply, it is of no use. Some managers believe that it is useful for "discipline" to keep staff a little nervous. Thus, these managers are slightly volatile and will be willing "to let them have it" when the situation demands. If you do this, you must be consistent and fair so that you staff know where they stand. **If you deliberately lose your temper for effect, then that is your decision - however, you must never lose control.**

Insults are ineffective. If you call people names, then they are unlikely to actually listen to what you have to say; in the short term you may feel some relief at "getting it off your chest", but in the long run you are merely perpetuating the problem since you are not addressing it. This is common sense. There are two implications. Firstly, even under pressure, you have to remember this. Secondly, what you consider fair comment may be insulting to another - and the same problem emerges. Before you say anything, stop, establish what you want as the outcome, plan how to achieve this, and then speak.

Finally, if you are going to criticise or discipline someone, always assume that you have misunderstood the situation and ask questions first which check the facts. This simple courtesy will save you from much embarrassment.

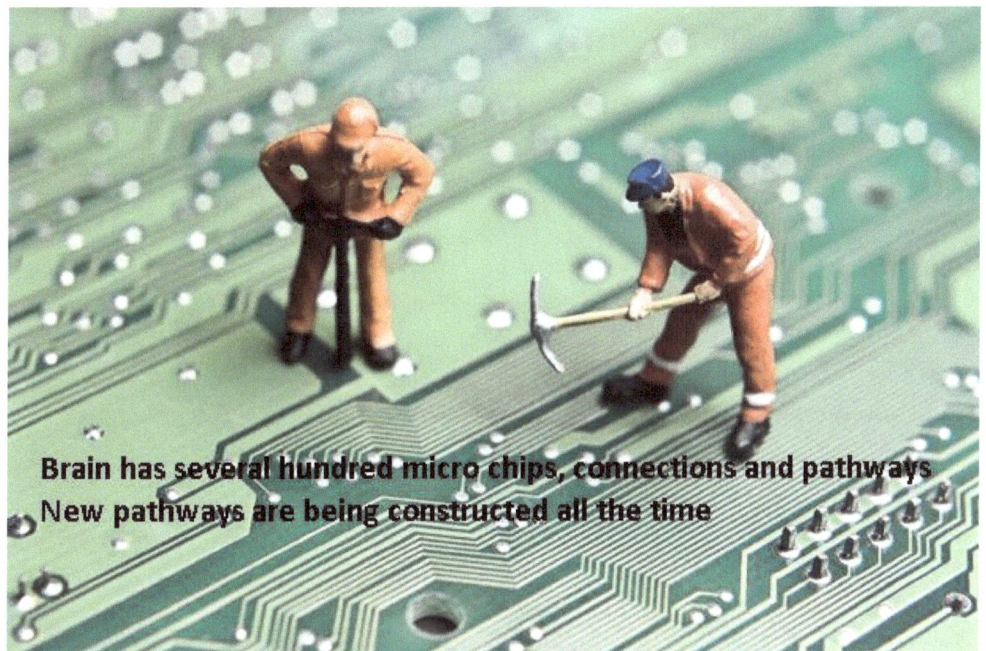

Brain has several hundred micro chips, connections and pathways New pathways are being constructed all the time

Questioning

Questioning is an important part of day to day communication and working. It helps appraisal of situation and can be used to subtle hints or suggestions. A careful questioning yields a lot more information and confidence in accuracy of information.

Asking the right question is at the heart of effective communications and information exchange. By using the right questions in a particular situation, you can improve a whole range of communications skills i.e. you can gather better information and learn more; you can build stronger relationships, manage people more effectively and help others to learn too.

There are two ways of phrasing any question: one way (the closed question) is likely to lead to a simple grunt in reply (yes, no, maybe), the second way (the open question) will hand over the speaking role to someone else and force them to say something a little more informative.

Open questions are good for developing an open conversation (how is your new job), finding out more detail (what else do we need to do to make this a success), finding out the other person's opinion or issues (what do you think about those changes).

Closed questions are good for testing understanding (your own or the other person's) i.e. " Did you say you can manage this project on your own?" It can also be used for concluding a discussion or making a decision or for general agreement (Now we know the facts, are we all agreed this is the right course of action?)

A misplaced closed question, on the other hand, can kill the conversation and lead to awkward silences, so are best avoided when a conversation is in full flow.

Asking probing questions is another strategy for finding out more detail. Sometimes it's as simple as asking your respondent for an example, to help you understand a statement they have made. At other times, you need additional information for clarification, "When do you need this report by, and do you want to see a draft before I give you my final version?", or to investigate whether there is proof for what has been said, "How do you know that the new database can't be used by the sales force?"

Q. Have you ever experience your questioning not giving you the desired information? What were the possible reasons and what you could have done to manage it better?

....

....

....

....

Q. How do you plan the informal appraisal of your projects?

....

....

....

....

Effective Communication in meetings

In any organization, "meetings" are a vital part of the organization of work and the flow of information. They act as a mechanism for gathering together resources from many sources and pooling then towards a common objective. They are disliked and mocked because they are usually futile, boring, time-wasting, dull, and inconvenient with nothing for most people to do except doodle while some opinionated has-been extols the virtues of his/her last great (misunderstood) idea. Your challenge is to break this mould and to make your meetings effective. As with every other managed activity, meetings should be planned beforehand, monitored during for effectiveness, and reviewed afterwards for improving their management.

A meeting is the ultimate form of managed conversation; as a manager, you can organize the information and structure of the meeting to support the effective communication of the participants. Some of the ideas below may seem a little too precise for an easy going, relaxed, semi-informal team atmosphere - but if you manage to gain a reputation for holding decisive, effective meetings, then people will value this efficiency and to prepare professionally so that their contribution will be heard.

Q. What efforts do you make for managing effective communication in meeting?

....

....

....

....

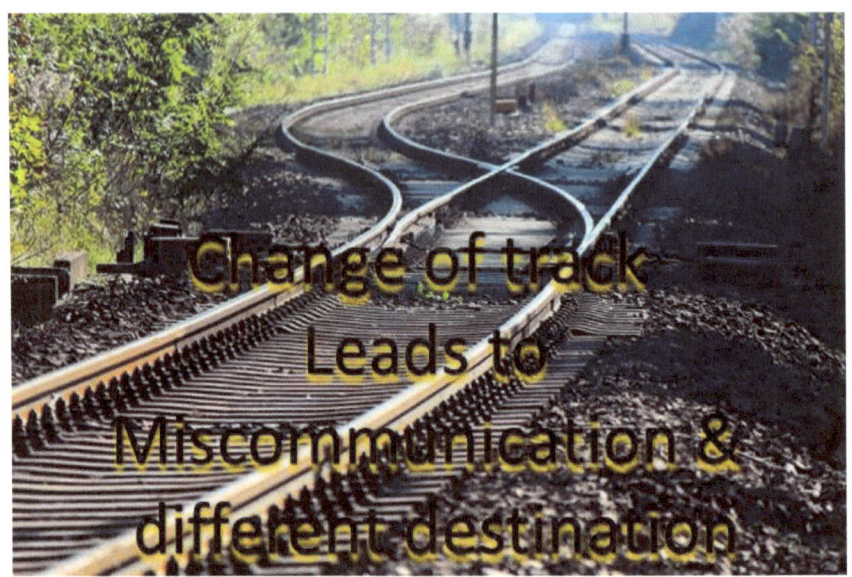

Change of track
Leads to
Miscommunication &
different destination

Effective Communication in meetings- PREPARATION

ASK questions to yourself before the meeting

Should you cancel?

As with all conversations, you must first ask: is it worth your time? If the meeting involves the interchange of views and the communication of the current status of related projects, then you should be generous with your time. But you should always consider cancelling a meeting which has little tangible value.

Who should attend?

You must be strict. A meeting loses its effectiveness if too many people are involved: so if someone has no useful function, explain this and suggest that they do not come. Notice, they may disagree with your assessment, in which case they should attend (since they may know something you do not); however, most people are only too happy to be released from yet another meeting.

How long?

It may seem difficult to predict the length of a discussion - but you must. Discussions tend to fill the available time which means that if the meeting is open-ended, it will drift on forever. You should stipulate a time for the end of the meeting so that everyone knows, and everyone can plan the rest of their day with confidence.

It is wise to make this expectation known to everyone involved well in advance and to remind them at the beginning of the meeting. There is often a tendency to view meetings as a little relaxation since no one person has to be active throughout. You can redress this view by stressing the time-scale and thus forcing the pace of the discussion: "this is what we have to achieve, this is how long we have to get it done".

If some unexpected point arises during the meeting then realize that since it is unexpected: 1) you might not have the right people present, 2) those there may not have the necessary information, and 3) a little thought might save a lot of discussion. If the new discussion looks likely to be more than a few moments, stop it and deal with the agreed agenda. The new topic should then be dealt with at another "planned" meeting.

Agenda

The purpose of an agenda is to inform participants of the subject of the meeting in advance, and to structure the discussion at the meeting itself. To inform people beforehand, and to solicit ideas, you should circulate a draft agenda and ask for notice of any other business. Still before the meeting, you should then send the revised agenda with enough time for people to prepare their contributions. If you know in advance that a particular participant either needs information or will be providing information, then make this explicitly clear so that there is no confusion.

The agenda states the purpose of each section of the meeting. There will be an outcome from each section. If that outcome is so complex that it can not be summarized in a few points, then it was probably too complex to be assimilated by the participants. The understanding of the meeting should be sufficiently precise that it can be summarized in short form - so display that summary for all other interested parties to see. This form of display will emphasize to all that meetings are about achieving defined goals - this will help you to continue running efficient meetings in the future.

Effective Communication in meetings- CONDUCTING

Whether you actually sit as the Chair or simply lead from the side-lines, as the manager you must provide the necessary support to coordinate the contributions of the participants. The degree of control which you exercise over the meeting will vary throughout; if you get the structure right at the beginning, a meeting can effectively run itself especially if the participants know each other well. In a team, your role may be partially undertaken by others; but if not, you must manage.

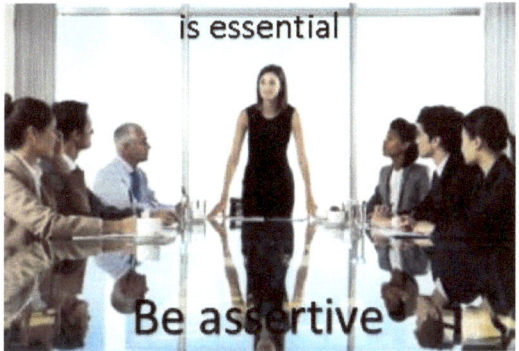

Your most important tools are:

- Clarification - always clarify: the purpose of the meeting, the time allowed, the rules to be observed (if agreed) by everyone.

- Summary - at each stage of the proceedings, you should summarize the current position and progress: this is what we have achieved/agreed, this is where we have reached.

- Focus on stated goals - at each divergence or pause, re-focus the proceedings on the original goals.

Code of conduct- In any meeting, it is possible to begin the proceedings by establishing a code of conduct, often by merely stating it and asking for any objections (which will only be accepted if a demonstrably better system is proposed). Thus if the group contains opinionated wind-bags, you might all agree at the onset that all contributions should be limited to two minutes (which focuses the mind admirably). You can then impose this with the full backing of the whole group.

Matching method to purpose- The (stated) purpose of a meeting may suggest to you a specific way of conducting the event, and each section might be conducted differently. For instance, if the purpose is:

o to convey information, the meeting might begin with a formal presentation followed by questions

o to seek information, the meeting would start with a short (clear) statement of the topic/problem and then an open discussion supported by notes on a display, or a formal brainstorming session

o to make a decision, the meeting might review the background and options, establish the criteria to be applied, agree who should make the decision and how, and then do it

o to ratify/explain decisions, etc

As always, once you have paused to ask yourself the questions: what is the purpose of the meeting and how can it be most effectively achieved; your common sense will then suggest a working method to expedite the proceedings. You just have to deliberately pause. Manage the process of the meeting and the meeting will work.

Support- The success of a meeting will often depend upon the confidence with which the individuals will participate. Thus all ideas should be welcome. No one should be laughed at or dismissed ("laughed with" is good, "laughed at" is destructive). This means that even bad ideas should be treated seriously - and at least merit a specific reason for not being pursued further. Not only is this supportive to the speaker, it could also be that a good idea has been misunderstood and would be lost if merely rejected. But basically people should be able to make naive contributions without being made to feel stupid, otherwise you may never hear the best ideas of all.

Avoid direct criticism of any person. For instance, if someone has not come prepared then that fault is obvious to all. If you leave the criticism as being simply that implicit in the peer pressure, then it is diffuse and general; if you explicitly rebuke that person, then it is personal and from you (which may raise unnecessary conflict). You should merely seek an undertaking for the missing preparation to be done: we need to know this before we can proceed, could you circulate it to us by tomorrow lunch?

Effective Communication in meetings- RESPONDING TO PROBLEMS

This section is devoted to ideas of how you might deal with the various problems associated with the volatile world of meetings. Some are best undertaken by the designated Chair; but if he/she is ineffective, or if no one has been appointed, you should feel free to help any meeting to progress. After all, why should you allow your time to be wasted?

If a participant strays from the agenda item, call him/her back: "we should deal with that separately, but what do you feel about the issue X?"

If there is confusion, you might ask: "do I understand correctly that ...?"

If the speaker begins to ramble, wait until an inhalation of breath and jump in: "yes I understand that such and such, does any one disagree?"

If a point is too woolly or too vague ask for greater clarity: "what exactly do you have in mind?"

If someone interrupts (someone other than a rambler), you should suggest that: " can we hear your contribution after Tom has finished."

If people chat, you might either simply state your difficulty in hearing/concentrating on the real speaker or ask them a direct question: "what do you think about that point." If you have set ground rules to respect all participants of meeting, remind them of that.

If someone gestures disagreement with the speaker (e.g. by a grimace), then make sure they are brought into the discussion next: "what do you think Anne?"

If you do not understand, say so: "I do not understand that, would you explain it a little more; or do you mean X or Y?"

If there is an error, look for a good point first: "I see how that would work if X Y Z, but what would happen if A B C?"

If you disagree, be very specific: "I disagree because ..."

Communicating (presenting) to large audience-1

It is becoming increasingly important to communicate to a group of stake holders or audience to present plan, convincing about a new project, or make them aware of the change. Leaders and mangers with good communication skills should be able to do it well, it just need tweaking skills so that you are reading body signals of many receivers in audience. Your message delivery need to be based on feedback keeping the main content still the same. When someone presents well, it sends the message that the person is capable, confident, intelligent, and competent. These people get noticed and that type of attention goes well for your career.

Preparation presenting to large audience

Tips to control nervousness

- o Calm yourself from the inside(it is Ok to be nervous, great presenters have been nervous)
- o Nervousness causes physiological reactions which are mostly attributed to the increase of adrenaline in your system. You can counteract these effects with a few simple techniques
- o Practice deep breathing - adrenalin causes you to breath shallowly. By breathing deeply your brain will get the oxygen it needs and the slower pace will trick your body into believing you are calmer. It also helps with voice quivers, which can occur when your breathing is irregular
- o Drink water - adrenalin can cause a dry mouth, which in turn leads to getting tongue-tied. Have a glass of water handy. Take sips occasionally, especially when you want to emphasize a point
- o Smile - this is a natural relaxant that sends positive chemicals through your body
- o Use visualization techniques - imagine that you are delivering your presentation to an audience that is interested, enthused, smiling, and reacting positively. Cement this positive image in your mind and recall it right before you are ready to go on;
- o Press and massage your forehead to bring to energize the front of the brain and speech centre
- o Just before you start talking, pause, make eye contact, and smile. This last moment of peace is very relaxing and gives you time to adjust to being the centre of attention
- o Speak more slowly than you would in a conversation, and leave longer pauses between sentences. This slower pace will calm you down, and it will also make you easier to hear, especially at the back of a large room
- o Move around during your presentation. This will expend some of your nervous energy
- o Stop Thinking About Yourself. Remember that the audience is there to get some information and it is your job to put it across to them.

Know Your Audience

Consult your audience before your presentation. The more confident you are that you are presenting them with useful and interesting material for them, the less nervous you will be overall. You really don't want your presentation to be a surprise. If it is, you lose complete control over the audience's reaction and that is a large factor in nervousness. So:
Define who your target audience is;
Ask people who are representative of the audience what they expect from the presentation;
Run your agenda by a few people to see if they think something is missing or is overkill;
Consider contacting participants by email beforehand and asking them a few questions about what they expect;
Greet audience members at the door and do a quick survey of why they are there and what they expect.

Prepare Your Material

Nothing is worse for nerves than trying to give a presentation on a topic you are not well prepared for. This doesn't mean you have to be an expert beforehand, but you'd better know it backwards on presentation day.

Prepare the structure of the talk carefully and logically, just as you would for a written report. What are the objectives of the talk? What are the main points you want to make?

Make a list of these two things as your starting point

Write out the presentation in rough, just like a first draft of a written report. Review the draft. You will find things that are irrelevant or superfluous - delete them. Check the story is consistent and flows smoothly. If there are things you cannot easily express, possibly because of doubt about your understanding, it is better to leave them unsaid.

Never read from a script. It is also unwise to have the talk written out in detail as a prompt sheet - the chances are you will not locate the thing you want to say amongst all the other text. You should know most of what you want to say - if you don't then you should not be giving the talk! So prepare cue cards which have key words and phrases (and possibly sketches) on them. Postcards are ideal for this. Don't forget to number the cards in case you drop them.

If you are using audio-visuals remember to mark on your cards the visual aids that go with them so that the right slide.

Practice presenting your talk

If it is a large audience presentation, rehearse your presentation - to yourself at first and then in front of some colleagues. The initial rehearsal should consider how the words and the sequence of visual aids go together.

Although you should avoid memorizing your presentation, you do want to be very comfortable with your delivery. Familiarity brings confidence, and practice helps you to deliver the words naturally. This means they will be coming more from your heart and mind, rather than from a piece of paper.

Learn the organization and order of your presentation;
If you do feel the need to memorize, limit it to your opening. This will help you get off to a smooth start;
Try videotaping yourself. You will see what you look like to others and then you can make a plan to change the things that need changing;
Use audiotape to listen to how you speak, your tone and your speed, and adjust appropriately;
Prepare for large speaking events by practicing with a smaller audience first; for example, by inviting colleagues to listen to a dry run during their lunch hour.

Delivering well

- Speak clearly. Don't shout or whisper - judge the acoustics of the room.

- Don't rush, or talk deliberately slowly. Be natural - although not conversational.

- Deliberately pause at key points - this has the effect of emphasising the importance of a particular point you are making.

- Avoid jokes unless you are a natural expert

- To make the presentation interesting, change your delivery i.e. speed and tone of voice

- Use your hands to emphasise points but don't indulge in to much hand waving. People can, over time, develop irritating habits. Ask colleagues occasionally what they think of your style.

- Look at the audience as much as possible, but don't fix on an individual - it can be intimidating. Pitch your presentation towards the back of the audience, especially in larger rooms.

- Don't face the display screen behind you and talk to it. Other annoying habits include:

   -Standing in a position where you obscure the screen. In fact, positively check for anyone in the audience who may be disadvantaged and try to accommodate them.
   -Muttering over a slide or transparency not realising that you are blocking the projection of the image.

Avoid moving about too much. Pacing up and down can unnerve the audience, although some animation is desirable.

Keep an eye on the audience's body language. Know when to stop and also when to cut out a piece of the presentation.

Your voice - how you say it is as important as what you say
- Body language is a subject in its own right and something about which you better pay utmost attention. In essence, your body movements , posture and gestures will continue to express what your attitudes and thoughts really are.
- Appearance - first impressions influence the audience's attitudes to you. Dress appropriately for the occasion. Decide what you are going to wear - make it comfortable and appropriate
- Arrive early and get your equipment set up if you are using a slide projector or other media for presentation.
- Anticipate problems and have backups and contingencies in place in case something doesn't work, you forget something, etc;
- If possible, give everything one last run through in the real environment;
- Prepare responses to anticipated questions. Try to think like that one person in the front row who always tries to trip the presenter up.

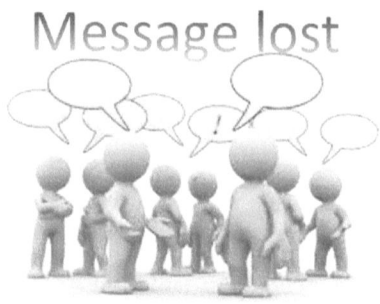

Message lost

Even if you don't make formal presentations in your current position, think about the future and keep in mind that you do have to present your ideas and opinions on a daily basis. The same basic principles of effective delivery apply.

Commonly it might not be to an audience of hundreds, but giving presentations to staff or even team members is a common enough occurrence. You owe it to yourself to develop some strategies and techniques to manage your nerves so you can concentrate on delivering an effective and engaging presentation.

Six Steps to Conquering Your Presentation Nerves

1. Know Your Audience-
    a. Consult your audience before your presentation. The more confident you are that you are presenting them with useful and interesting material for them; the less nervous you will be overall. You really don't want your presentation to be a surprise. If it is, you lose complete control over the audience's reaction and that is a large factor in nervousness. So:
    b. Define who your target audience is;
    c. Ask people who are representative of the audience what they expect from the presentation;
    d. Run your agenda by a few people to see if they think something is missing or is overkill;
    e. Consider contacting participants by email beforehand and asking them a few questions about what they expect;
    f. Greet audience members at the door and do a quick survey of why they are there and what they expect.
2. Know Your Material-
    a. Nothing is worse for nerves than trying to give a presentation on a topic you are not well prepared for. This doesn't mean you have to be an expert beforehand, but you'd better know it backwards on presentation day. And making sure you've understood

your audience and their needs properly will help you ensure that your material is on target to meet their needs.

b. Another important point to remember is that you can't possibly cover everything you know in your presentation. That would probably be long and boring. So select the most pertinent points from your subject base and then supplement with other material if time allows.

3. Structure Your Presentation

A common technique for trying to calm nervousness is memorizing what you intend to say (not the detailed content). But all this does is make your delivery sound like it is coming from a robot. If you miss a word or draw a blank, your whole presentation is thrown off and then your nervousness compounds itself with every remaining second. It is far better to structure your presentation so that you give yourself clues to what is coming next.

- Have a set of key phrases listed on a cue card;
- Refer to these phrases to trigger your mind as to what is coming up next;
- If you're using slides, use these key phrases in your transitions.

This approach helps you control your own uncertainty about whether you will remember what you want to say and the order you want to say it.

4. Practice, Practice, Practice
Although you should avoid memorizing your presentation, you do want to be very comfortable with your delivery. Familiarity brings confidence, and practice helps you to deliver the words naturally. This means they will be coming more from your heart and mind, rather than from a piece of paper.
Learn the organization and order of your presentation;
If you do feel the need to memorize, limit it to your opening. This will help you get off to a smooth start;
Try videotaping yourself. You will see what you look like to others and then you can make a plan to change the things that need changing;
Use audiotape to listen to how you speak, your tone and your speed, and adjust appropriately;
Prepare for large speaking events by practicing with a smaller audience first; for example, by inviting colleagues to listen to a dry run during their lunch hour.

Standing near podium to show slides and looking at data projected rather than audience is not uncommon. In fact that is how most presentations are delivered, but this kind of presentation risks boring your audience to the point where they are either going to sleep or waiting for a fire alarm to go off so they can escape. And once you lose someone, it is next to impossible to bring his or her attention back.

If the information you are presenting is important enough for you to deliver orally, then it demands an appropriate amount of planning and preparation so that the information you present is memorable – for the right reasons. You need to deliver the information in different headings and in form of bullet points on slide. You however need to know majority of important data in presentation. If that is important to your audience, it is important that you have a grasp of the details (may not need to memorise the details).

Commonly presenters ignore looking to audience which actually prevent a good delivery. The common reason is anxiety or stage fright.

Give a bad presentation and you'll be remembered all right: It just won't be the type of impression you want to leave in anyone's mind.

Communicating in a crisis situation

When a crisis or some other adverse situation occurs, the natural instinct is to close ranks, work furiously to contain the damage, and set the situation back to normal. We go into protection mode – for both our organization and ourselves.

However this approach can badly wrong. We've all seen major companies terribly wounded when the press senses a "cover up." And we may also have seen situations where gossip has spiralled out of control with damaging results. When official communication channels are shut down, communication does not stop. In fact it can often increase wildly.

Few important hints

- Don't shut down communication
- Have a single line of commands
- Give a clear concise message
- If problem has occurred, Don't hide facts
- Accept mistakes possibly without naming and shaming the person responsible
- Focus on next action and timing
- If specific teams or sub-groups need different actions, designate specifically
- Deliver your messages calmly and confidently

The problem is that this communication can be full of rumour, innuendo, inconsistencies, half truths, and exaggerations. More than this, the trust and confidence of employees and clients can be undermined, with often-damaging long term consequences.

Q. Have you ever faced crisis in your professional or personal life and what did you learn from it?

....

....

....

....

Emotions in communication

Emotion is an extremely important content of communication. Successful leaders or managers are very good at identifying and responding to emotions of others. Emotional intelligence is gaining popularity in leaders, executives and managers.

Paul Ekman in mid 1960s studied emotions and discovered six facial expressions that almost everyone recognizes world-wide: happiness, sadness, anger, fear, disgust, and surprise. One of the controversies still lingering is the amount of context needed to interpret them. For example, if someone reports to me that they have this great idea to increase that they would like to implement to increase income, and I say that would be great, but I look on them with a frown; is it possible that I could be thinking about something else or I dislike the idea but have no choice to stop him? The trouble with these extra signals is that we do not always have the full context. What if the person emailed me and I replied great (while frowning). Would it evoke the same response?

The other aspect is managing your own emotions. Trust your instincts. Most emotions are difficult to imitate. For example, when you are truly happy, the muscles used for smiling are controlled by the limbic system and other parts of the brain, which are not under voluntary control. When you force a smile, a different part of the brain is used - the cerebral cortex (under voluntary control), hence different muscles are used. This is why a clerk, who might not have any real interest in you, has a "fake" look when he forces a smile.

Of course, some actors learn to control all of their face muscles, while others draw on a past emotional experience to produce the emotional state they want. But this is not an easy trick to pull off all the time. There is a good reason for this - part of our emotions evolved to deal with other people and our empathic nature.

If these emotions could easily be faked, they would do more harm than good (Pinker, 1997).

So our emotions not only guide our decisions, they can also be communicated to others to help them in their decisions - of course their emotions will be the ultimate guide, but the emotions they discover in others become part of their knowledge base.

Q what is your view on value of emotions in communication?

....

....

....

....

Q. How do you identify and manage unwanted emotions in your professional or personal life?

....

....

....

....

Communication research Albert Mehrabian

Mehrabian and the 7%-38%-55% Myth

We often hear that the content of a message is composed of:

- 55% from the visual component
- 38% from the auditory component
- 7% from language

However, the above percentages only apply in a very narrow context. A researcher named Mehrabian was interested in how listeners get their information about a speaker's general attitude in situations where the facial expression, tone, and/or words are sending conflicting signals.

Thus, he designed a couple of experiments. In one, Mehrabian and Ferris (1967) researched the interaction of speech, facial expressions, and tone. Three different speakers were instructed to say "maybe" with three different attitudes towards their listener (positive, neutral, or negative). Next, photographs of the faces of three female models were taken as they attempted to convey the emotions of like, neutrality, and dislike.

Test groups were then instructed to listen to the various renditions of the word "maybe," with the pictures of the models, and were asked to rate the attitude of the speaker. Note that the emotion and tone were often mixed, such as a facial expression showing dislike, with the word "maybe" spoken in a positive tone.

Significant effects of facial expression and tone were found in that the study suggested that the combined effect of simultaneous verbal, vocal and facial attitude communications is a weighted sum of their independent effects with the coefficients of .07, .38, and .55, respectively.

Mehrabian and Ferris also wrote about a deep limitation to their research: "These findings regarding the relative contribution of the tonal component of a verbal message can be safely extended only to communication situations in which no additional information about the communicator-addressee relationship is available." Thus, what can be concluded is that when people communicate, listeners derive information about the speaker's attitudes towards the listener from visual, tonal, and verbal cues; yet the percentage derived can vary greatly depending upon a number of other factors, such as actions, context of the communication, and how well they know that person.

Quantum Physics and communication

EVERYTHING at it's core consists of pure energy and EVERYTHING, both the seen (physical) and the unseen (metaphysical) is intricately interconnected with EVERYTHING else at this level of causation which is a continuously vibrating mass of pure energy.

Bio-cabinets for thoughts

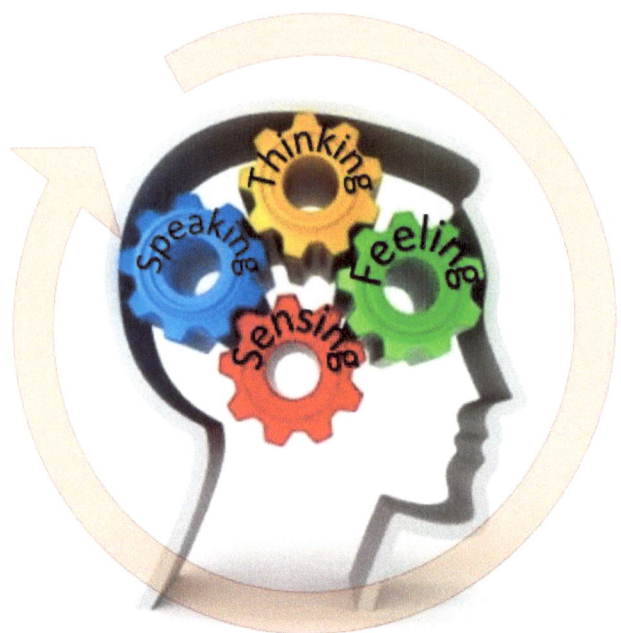

NLP model for communication and filtering

NLP (Nero Linguistic Programming) is the most widely accepted tool utilized today for producing rapid results. It is actually a collection of models of how we as humans produce and create our reality. Yes, we create our reality because reality isn't what is going on outside of us, but rather what is going on inside of us. For many, that's almost completely opposite from what we have been taught or learned throughout our entire lives.

Our minds (somewhat like a computer) operate or run on programs. These human programs have been gathering and storing information our entire lives. These programs consist of our language, attitudes, beliefs, values, emotions, memories, etc. (see diagram). And, just like a computer, occasionally these 'programs' may become obsolete or develop a glitch and need to be reformatted or updated (especially when there is some type of difficulty or problem).

If you are wanting to make a change and want that change to come as rapidly as possible and if your time is important and you're not willing to invest months or even years in obtaining that change, then NLP and hypnosis may be right for you.

This model is a way of explaining how we take information from the outside world into our neurology and how that in turn affects our behaviours.

The process begins with an external event which enters our nervous system through the five senses that make up our sensory input channels:-

- **Visual** - what we see
- **Auditory** - sound, the words we hear and how those words are said to us etc.
- **Kinaesthetic** - internal and external feelings, pressure, texture etc.
- **Olfactory** - the sense of smell
- **Gustatory** - the sense of taste

These sensory input channels are often referred to in NLP by their initial letters - **V,A, K, O** and **G** respectively.

The NLP communication model includes the notion that our five senses take in up to 2,000,000 (two million) bits of information per second. The notion further states that our conscious mind can only process 7+/-2* chunks of information per second which equates to approximately 134 bits per second. It doesn't take a math degree to see that our fantastic senses make available far more information than the conscious mind can usefully cope with - so what happens to the rest?

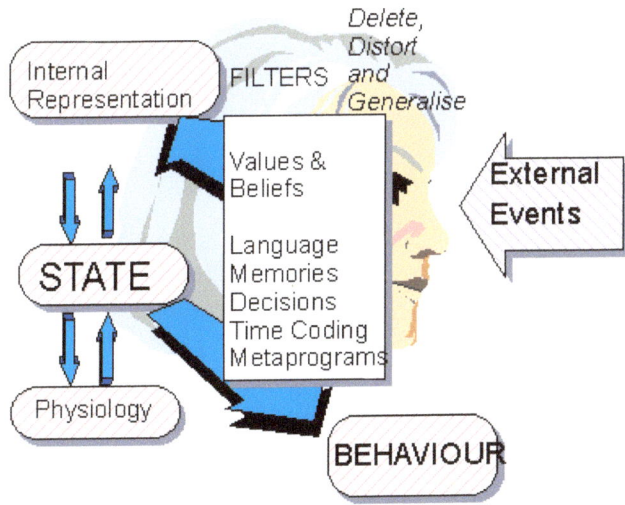

The incoming information passes automatically through a number of filters to reduce the information down to the 7+/2* chunks or (roughly) 134 bits that our conscious mind can cope with. The filters do this by:-

Deletion - to attempt to actively pay attention to everything entering though our sensory input channels would not be useful. Thus we omit certain parts of our current experience by selectively paying attention to certain other parts of it i.e. we focus on what seems most important at any one particular moment in time and allow the rest to pass us by.

A common example of why deletion is necessary is that of the use of mobile telephones whilst driving - statistics prove that so much information is deleted when we try to do these two tasks simultaneously that we end up doing both badly and sometimes with very serious consequences.

Distortion - occurs when we make shifts in our experience of sensory data by making misrepresentations of reality. Distortion is a key component of imagination and a useful tool in motivating ourselves toward our goals. When we plan we use distortion to construct appealing imaginary futures.

As another example ask yourself a simple question - would you recognise your best friend if they changed their clothes or styled their hair in a different way? Without the ability to distort reality the answer would be no. Every time your friend changed a single aspect of their appearance, hair length, hair colour, clothing type, clothing colour etc., you would have to learn that entire configuration and add it to the 'map' which you label 'my best friend'.

Each time you saw your friend the only way you could be sure it was them would be to mentally examine every 'version' of them in the map until you found one that matched the person standing in front of you. Add in the fact that they look different depending on their facial expression, physical posture, state of health etc., etc. and the number of combinations you would have to learn just to recognise your friend would be huge! If you have more than one friend then you really have your work cut out for you!

Thus we rely on distortion to allow us to identify a particular thing or person over a wide range of variance.

The example in the Presuppositions section for feeling less stressed during a job interview by picturing the interviewer in the nude is also a good example of distortion.

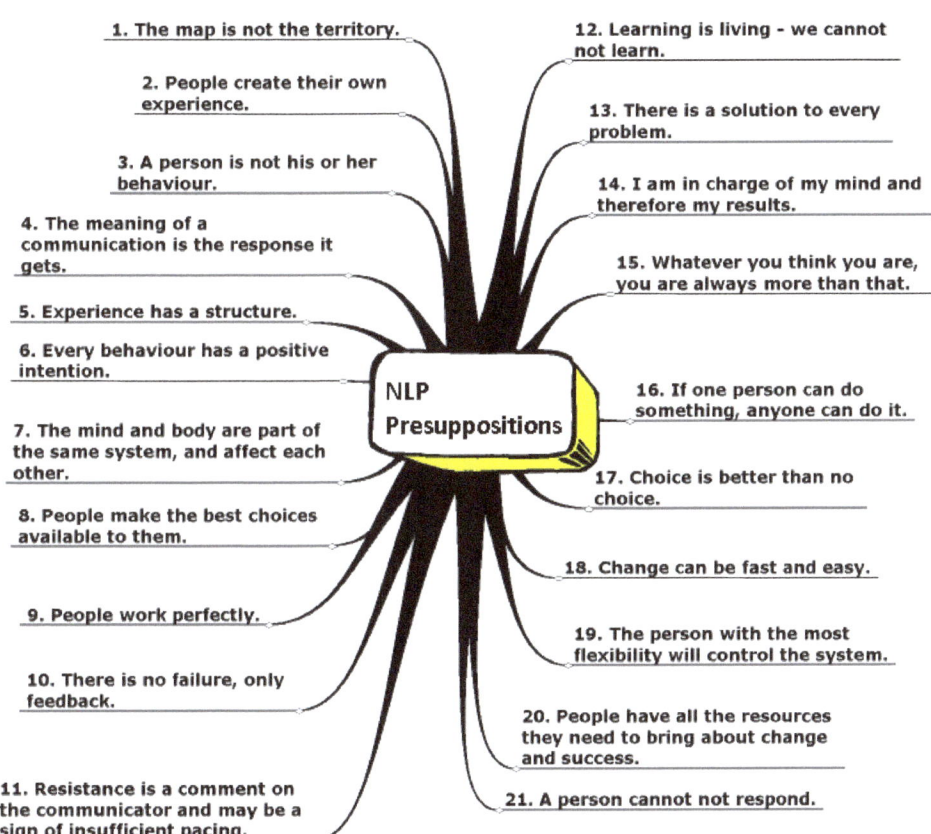

NLP Presuppositions

1. The map is not the territory.
2. People create their own experience.
3. A person is not his or her behaviour.
4. The meaning of a communication is the response it gets.
5. Experience has a structure.
6. Every behaviour has a positive intention.
7. The mind and body are part of the same system, and affect each other.
8. People make the best choices available to them.
9. People work perfectly.
10. There is no failure, only feedback.
11. Resistance is a comment on the communicator and may be a sign of insufficient pacing.
12. Learning is living - we cannot not learn.
13. There is a solution to every problem.
14. I am in charge of my mind and therefore my results.
15. Whatever you think you are, you are always more than that.
16. If one person can do something, anyone can do it.
17. Choice is better than no choice.
18. Change can be fast and easy.
19. The person with the most flexibility will control the system.
20. People have all the resources they need to bring about change and success.
21. A person cannot not respond.

Generalisation - is the process by which we draw global conclusions based on one, two or more experiences.

A useful example of a generalisation is that of a door. We learn that a door is usually a conduit between two locations - an exit from one location and simultaneously an entry into another location. We also learn that most doors are fixed along one side about an axis of rotation and that if we pull or push on the opposite side of the door it will open in one direction and close in the other. This is a superbly efficient form of learning as once we've learned how one door works we have the necessary information to deal with doors of any colour, size, shape or composition in any location so long as they conform to that basic type and we can commit this information to memory for future use.

At it's best generalisation is an efficient means of learning information which can be applied globally. At it's worst it is the way we take a single event and turn it into a lifetime of experience i.e. most phobias arise as a result of a one-time learning.

*7+/-2 (seven plus or minus two) represents the number of chunks of information that the conscious mind can usefully attend to at any point in time. To clarify, in optimum conditions i.e. calm, relaxed, quiet, focussed, an average person could attend to up to 9 chunks of information at any one time. Under less than ideal conditions i.e. noisy, stressed and distracted by other things, an

average person may only be able to attend to 5 chunks of information at any one time. Most of the time the average person can attend to 7 chunks of information at any one time.

Chunk size is variable and usually relates to the complexity of each chunk. Further explanations relating to chunking can be found elsewhere on this website.

Learning about the the individual sensory filters and how they delete, distort and generalise the information coming in through our five senses will be covered on the next page. For now it's more useful to close the loop on the NLP communication model by explaining what happens to the information once it has passed through the filters, providing the resultant 7+/-2 chunks or 134 bits of data that the conscious mind can usefully attend to.

So far the data from the external event - the sights, sounds, feelings, tastes and smells, has been filtered down to a manageable size. This data then gets stored in our mind as an internal representation of that external event. How that internal representation (IR) compares with the external event will depend on what the filters deleted, how the filters distorted the data and whether any existing or freshly made generalisations were applied.

It's also worth noting at this stage that generalisations can get revised as we make new learnings and these revisions can cause us to re-evaluate internal representations we've made about past external events i.e. we see things in a new light and have a different appreciation / change our opinions of something that happened in the past. Remember - all learning and behaviour is geared towards adaptation.

So we have an internal representation (or thought if you prefer a 'user friendly' term) of an external event. That internal representation and our evaluation of it is intimately linked to our emotional state (how we feel), our physiology (body position, skin colour and temperature, muscle tone etc.) and to our behaviour (our actions) for example:-

- *Queueing for the latest big-thrill super-looping gut wrenching roller-coaster ride at our favourite theme park we see the train flash past, hear riders screaming, feel the vibrations resonate through the structure under the G-force. We may feel excited, feel the effects of adrenaline on our body and whoop with excitement as we push to the front of the queue. On the other hand we may feel sick with dread, attempt to make ourselves as small as possible and then run in the opposite direction as fast as our now wobbly legs can carry us.*

- *Hearing a pitiful 'miow' we look up to see a tiny kitten, successful in it's first adventure into tree climbing. Problem is that it hasn't worked out how to get down yet and it's cries suggest that it's none too pleased about it. We may feel sympathy for the tiny creature, adopt the persona of our favourite super hero and rescue this brave fur ball from it's predicament. On the other hand we may feel disdain for it's 'obvious stupidity', snarl in it's general direction decide that it should have thought about how it was going to get down from the tree before embarking on it's ascent and that it 'has to learn some time'.*

Now that we've considered two possible external events and seen how subjectively we could experience very different emotional states, experience very different changes in our physiology and exhibit very different behaviours we understand the beginning and end points of the NLP communication model.

The 'bits-in-the-middle' that influence which set or combination of state and physiology we will experience and which behaviours that might produce are the filters.

So now we understand that an external event passes through perceptual filters which delete, distort and generalise the incoming data, leaving a package of data that we can usefully attend to consciously. We also understand that our conscious mind stores that data in an internal representation (or memory) of that external event which is intimately linked with our emotional state and physiology which in turn influences our behaviours.

The perceptual filters that perform the deletion, distortion and generalisation processes are organised in layers thus:-

Meta Programs - are the most unconscious of the perception filters and are content free i.e. they are not based on any past experience or beliefs. Whether you see the glass as half empty or half full is an example of one of your meta programs.

Values - are the next most unconscious filter and are the first level at which the filters have content as they are based upon our experiences to date. Values are those things we are prepared to fight for and also those things we try to live up to. Values are those things we are prepared to invest resources in to either achieve or avoid. Values are how we know right from wrong, good from bad, what's important and what isn't, and they are also how we decide about how we feel about our actions and the actions of others.

Values are arranged in a hierarchy, usually with most important one at the top and the lesser ones below. Values are also context dependent - your values about what's important to you in a relationship are probably very different from you values about what's important to you in your career. Values can also be linked to and vary with changes in emotional state.

Beliefs - on one level beliefs are convictions that certain things are true or real and are also generalisations about the state of the world around us. Beliefs are presuppositions that we have about certain things and can create or deny personal power for us i.e. we have a better chance of achieving an objective if we first truly believe we are capable of doing so. If we believe that we will fail then the likelihood of that being our outcome increases. In modelling an ability we admire in another individual and desire for ourselves, finding out what the enabling beliefs are that allow that person to have that ability is vital.

Attitudes - are collections of values and beliefs around a particular subject. Often we are quite conscious of our attitudes and often we share them with others i.e. 'Well that's the way I feel about.....'. Change made at the level of attitude is far more difficult to achieve than change made at the level of values.

Memories - the collection of memories we build up during the course of our lives deeply affect both our perceptions and our personality. Our memories are who we are. Some psychologists believe that as we get older our reactions to present external events actually have very little to do with the present, and are in fact reactions to gestalts - collections of past memories organised in a certain way around certain subjects. Gestalts are formed when a number of individual experiences of the same type get squashed together to form one single generalised memory.

Decisions - the sixth filter, also related to memories are decisions which we made in our past. Decisions about who we are and what we are capable of, especially negative or limiting decisions, can affect our entire lives. The decisions we make may generate beliefs, values and attitudes or they may just affect our perceptions though time.

Sometimes we make decisions unconsciously or at a very early age and then forget them. These decisions may not get re-evaluated in the context of new experience and as a result can affect our lives in ways which were not originally intended.

Therapeutic uses of communication

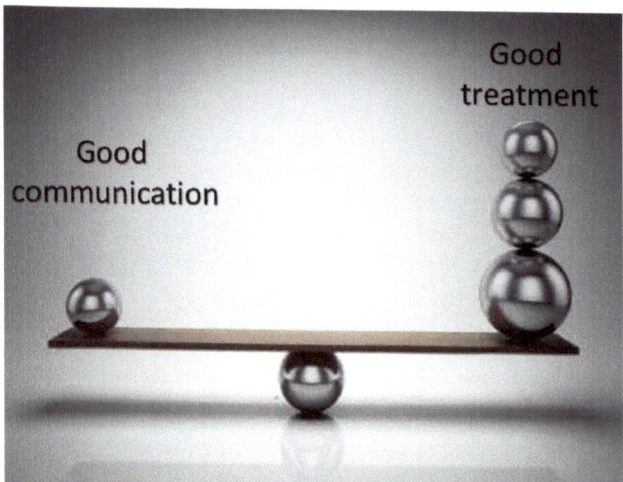

Using silence for communication is sometimes very powerful.
Other things to think about are

Using silence for communication

Intra-personal communication

Verbal conditioning

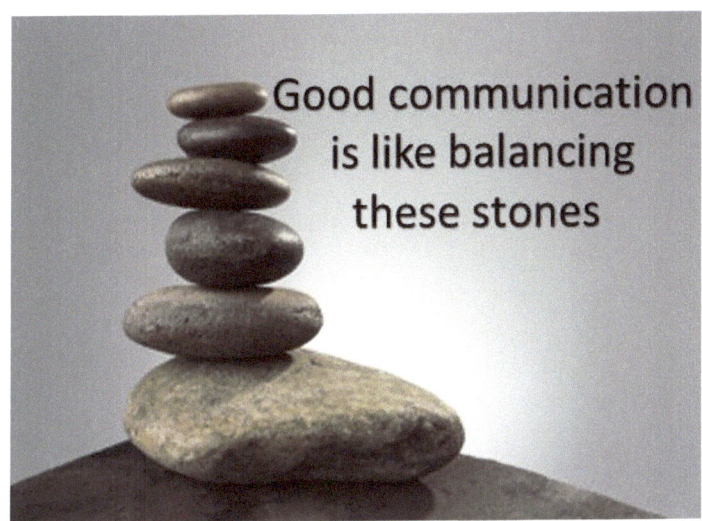

Good communication is like balancing these stones

Five tips for better communication

1. **Be clear and direct**. Majority of patient complaints are due to miscommunication, often not being clear. It is something that can be avoided and fixed by being conscious and clear in our own head of what is the message we want to give. To avoid confusion, it is good to look them in the eye, focus on the conversation at hand, and don't talk while you're engaged in something else.

2. **Say the person's name**. Before you begin a conversation, say the person's name so the listener has a better chance to focus their attention. This technique also reduces the chance of missing words at the beginning of a conversation. Having been addressed by name is said to increase retention of information.

3. **Avoid jargon**. Apart from mumbling, medical jargon is a constant barrier to good communication. The message is often lost as they start second guessing and unable to concentrate for next few minutes. Simple English campaign may be instructive.

4. **Be calm and composed**. Believe it or not, calmness bring confidence in talking. Remember to speak plainly and humbly. Be aware of your ticks and mannerisms. If your normal is a little rapid, be sure to slow the pace down a little.

5. **Check out what was heard**. Although it may sound pedantic, miscommunication can only be avoided by checking out that listener has got the message you wanted to give. You can say, I just wanted to check that I have communicated the right message. A good focus on body language of the listener or patient will give you a clue during the conversation that your message is filtering through.

References

Butler, Gillian, Ph.D. and Hope, Tony, M.D. (1996). Managing Your Mind. New York: Oxford University Press.

Mehrabian, Albert and Morton Wiener, 1967, "Decoding of inconsistent communications," Journal of Personality and Social Psychology 6:109-114

Mehrabian, Albert and Susan R. Ferris, 1967, "Inference of attitudes from nonverbal communication in two channels," Journal of Consulting Psychology 31:248-252.

Pearson, J. (1983). Interpersonal Communication. Glenview, Illinois: Scott, Foreman and Company.

Pinker, Steven (1997). How the Mind Works. New York: W. W. Norton & Company.